Visionaries from Lviv
The Story of
a Jewish Hospital

Jews of Poland

Series Editor
Antony Polonsky (Brandeis University)

Other Titles in this Series

Shaping the Jewish Enlightenment: Solomon Dubno (1738–1813),
an Eastern European Maskil
Zuzanna Krzemień
Edited by Noëmie Duhaut and Wojciech Tworek, in collaboration with Monika Biesaga

I Came Home and There Was No One There: Conversations and Stories about the Uprising
in the Warsaw Ghetto
Hanka Grupińska
Translated from Polish by Jessica Taylor-Kucia

Leonid Hurwicz: Intelligent Designer: How War and the Great Depression
Inspired a Nobel Economist
Michael Hurwicz

A Man of Success in the Land of Success: The Biography of Marcel Goldman,
a Kracovian in Tel Aviv
Łukasz Tomasz Sroka
Translated by Katarzyna Rogalska-Chodecka

Polish Jews in the Soviet Union (1939–1959): History and Memory of Deportation,
Exile, and Survival
Edited by Katharina Friedla and Markus Nesselrodt

Bolesław Prus and the Jews
Agnieszka Friedrich
Translated by Ben Koschalka

Visionaries from Lviv

The Story of a Jewish Hospital

Ewa Herbst, Editor

BOSTON
2024

Library of Congress Control Number: 2024942998

ISBN 9798887192543 (hardcover)
ISBN 9798887194479 (Adove PDF)
ISBN 9798887194486 (ePub)

Copyright © 2024 Academic Studies Press.
All rights reserved

Academic consultant: Dr. habil. Anna Jakimyszyn-Gadocha

Book design by Lapiz Digital Services
Cover design by Kalina Paszyńska with Ivan Grave

On the cover: Jewish Hospital ca 1925. Photograph by Marek Münz.

Published by Academic Studies Press
1577 Beacon St., Brookline, MA 02446
press@academicstudiespress.com
www.academicstudiespress.com

The publication of this book was supported by
Furthermore: a program of the J. M. Kaplan Fund
and Gesher Galicia

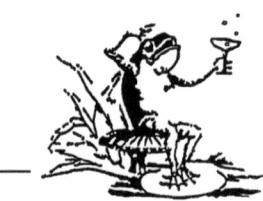

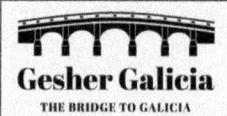

Contents

Acknowledgements — vii
Note on Place-Names and Terms — ix
Archives and Libraries — xi
Preface — xiii

1. Jewish Medical Practitioners from Galicia: Barber-Surgeons, Physicians, and Societal Trailblazers — 1
   Andrew Zalewski

2. Maurycy Lazarus, Founder of the Jewish Hospital, and His Family — 42
   Ewa Herbst

3. The Jewish Hospital in Lemberg/Lwów/Lviv: Its Architecture and Architects — 90
   Sergey R. Kravtsov

4. The Maurycy Lazarus Foundation Israelite Hospital (1903–1939) — 125
   Anna Jakimyszyn-Gadocha

Postscript — 154
Contributors — 156
Index — 158

Acknowledgements

There are many people to whom we are indebted for their support in the preparation of this book. We are grateful to Prof. Antony Polonsky for his interest in the topic and his early support. Several others are listed in respective chapters of the book.

The generous support of Furthermore (a program of the J. M. Kaplan Fund), Gesher Galicia, and private sponsors made the publication of this book possible. Ukrainian Jewish Encounter was instrumental in bringing additional support. Gesher Galicia, which is devoted to carrying out Jewish genealogical and historical research and promoting education about Galician Jewish culture and heritage, also sponsored the medical students research project that yielded rich archival material invaluable for the preparation of Chapter 1.

Chapter 2, about Maurycy Lazarus and his family, was strengthened by family stories collected by Halina Diamand-Stankiewicz, granddaughter of Maurycy Lazarus. They also created a springboard for further explorations.

Chapter 3 is based on Dr. Sergey Kravtsov's presentation at the conference "Ukrainian Jewish Encounter: Cultural Interaction, Representation and Memory," organized by the Ukrainian Jewish Encounter Initiative in collaboration with the Israel Museum and the Hebrew University of Jerusalem in October 2010, and his article "The Israelite Hospital in Lemberg/Lwów/Lviv, 1898–1912: 'Jewish' Architecture by an 'International' Team," *Jews and Slavs* 25 (2016). We are grateful to Alti Rodal and Prof. Wolf Moskovich, the editors of *Jews and Slavs*, for their endorsement of the present publication.

We would like to thank Prof. Łukasz T. Sroka and Prof. Christoph Mick for their comments on Chapter 4, as well as all individuals and institutions which made their collections and illustrations available to the authors.

Note on Place-Names and Terms

Note on Place-Names

Following the First Partition of Poland in 1772 between Russia, Austria (the Habsburg Monarchy), and Prussia, the region called Galicia, with Lviv as its capital, fell under the Habsburgs' reign. The territory of the Habsburg Monarchy, separate from the Holy Roman Empire nominally ruled by the Habsburgs at the time, was also referred to as the Austrian Monarchy. It became the Austrian Empire in 1804 and the Austro-Hungarian Empire in 1867, and those names are reflected in *Visionaries from Lviv: The Story of a Jewish Hospital*. Sometimes the term Habsburg Monarchy is used in literature for the whole Austrian period, as on one occasion in Chapter 3.

After the Partition of Poland, Polish Lwów became Lemberg (in German) and Lwów again by the end of the nineteenth century; and it stayed this way during the interwar Second Polish Republic. After World War II, when Poland's eastern border was redrawn, it became part of the Soviet Union as Lvov and then part of free Ukraine as L'viv. All contributors to this book have their family roots in the city, and their original texts contained two different spellings of the city's name. In the end, we decided to use the English spelling, Lviv, as it is the most recognized name today. We have tried to consistently use the English spelling of place-names, where they exist, with the old Polish and current Ukrainian names in parenthesis. The exception is Kraków, where we have used the original Polish spelling. Where there is no English name, we have used the Polish one (as the book talks about the period before World War II), with the current Ukrainian name in parenthesis, if different.

In the bibliography and notes we have made an exception to the above rule, giving the name Lwów or Lviv for the places of publishing houses. If publication took place before

World War II, we use Lwów; if it is a recent publication, we have Lviv. This indicates that the books were published in different countries (even if in the same city) and may contain different perspectives.

Names of the city suburbs may be confusing to the reader and require an explanation. The city of Lviv had four historical suburbs, which later became city districts of greater Lviv. They were: Halicz (Halych) suburb to the south, Kraków suburb to the west (in the direction of Kraków), Żółkiew (Zhovkva) suburb to the north, and Łyczaków (Lychakiv) suburb to the east.

Note on Terms

"Lazarus Jewish Hospital," or simply "Jewish Hospital" (as it is popularly known), refers to the Maurycy Lazarus Foundation Israelite Hospital, while "Jewish hospital" is used as a generic term.

The term "Jewish Community" is used in the text as synonymous with the official representation of the Jewish population (Israelitische Kultusgemeinde in German), while "Jewish community" (not capitalized) refers to the Jewish population of a given town. "Jewish Community Council" refers to an advisory body of the local Jewish Community.

Archives and Libraries

AAN, Archiwum Akt Nowych, New Records Archive, Warsaw, Poland

AGAD, Archiwum Główne Akt Dawnych, Central Archive of Historical Records, Warsaw, Poland

ANK, Archiwum Narodowe w Krakowie, National Archives in Kraków, Poland

APL, Archiwum Państwowe w Lublinie, State Archive in Lublin, Poland

APP, Archiwum Państwowe w Przemyślu, State Archive in Przemyśl, Poland

Archives Nationales de France, French National Archives, France

AUJ, Archiwum Uniwersytetu Jagiellońskiego, Jagiellonian University Archives, Kraków, Poland

BJ, Biblioteka Jagiellońska, Jagiellonian University Library, Kraków, Poland

BN, Biblioteka Narodowa, National Library of Poland, Warsaw, Poland

Center For Urban History, Lviv, Ukraine

DALO, Derzhavnyi Arkhiv L'vivs'koi oblasti, Lviv, State Archive of Lviv Oblast, Lviv, Ukraine

Digital Archives in Opava, Státní okresní archiv Opava, State District Archives in Opava, Opava, Czech Republic

Family Search: www.familysearch.org

Gesher Galicia, All Galicia Database: www.geshergalicia.org/all-galicia-database

HDA, Hrvatski državni arhiv, Croatian State Archives, Zagreb, Croatia

IKG, der Israelitischen Kultusgemeinde Wien Archiv, Archive of the Jewish Community of Vienna, Vienna, Austria

Institut Pasteur/Musée Pasteur, Paris, France

Jewish Museum, Berlin, Germany

Korczakianum, Muzeum Warszawy, Museum of Warsaw, Warsaw, Poland

LNNBU, L'vivs'ka natsional'na naukova biblioteka Ukrainy imeni Vasylia Stefanyka, Vasyl Stefanyk National Scientific Library of Ukraine in Lviv, Ukraine

NLI, National Library of Israel

NYPL, The New York Public Library, New York, USA

ÖNB, Österreichische Nationalbibliothek, Austrian National Library, Vienna, Austria

Ossolineum, Zakład Narodowy im. Ossolińskich, Ossoliński National Institute, Wrocław, Poland

ÖStA, Österreichisches Staatsarchiv, Austrian State Archive, Vienna, Austria

OSZK, Országos Széchényi Könyvtár, National Széchényi Library, Budapest, Hungary

PAU, Polska Akademia Umiejętności, Polish Academy of Arts and Sciences, Kraków, Poland

POLONA, The National Digital Library, Poland

SEL, Semmelweis Egyetem Levéltára, Semmelweis University Archives, Budapest, Hungary

TsDIAL, Tsentral'nyi derzhavnyi istorychnyi arkhiv Ukrainy, Lviv, Central State Historical Archives of Ukraine in Lviv, Ukraine

UAW, Wien Universitätsarchiv, Vienna University Archives, Austria

Wien Museum, Vienna Museum, Vienna, Austria

WSTLA, Wiener Stadt- und Landesarchiv, Vienna City and Provincial Archives, Vienna, Austria

Preface

The idea of this book was born in Lviv in June 2019 during my first visit to the city. While visiting the former Jewish Hospital, founded by my great-grandfather Maurycy Lazarus and still active today as a municipal maternity hospital, Dr. Oksana Mykoliv-Stadnyk, who made arrangements for my visit there, suggested that a book about the hospital would be an excellent way to mark its upcoming 120th anniversary in 2023. I returned to Lviv in December of 2019 to further discuss it with her and Iryna Kotlobulatova, a leading authority on the photographic history of Lviv. Soon after my visit, however, the pandemic immobilized the world. Time passed, but the idea of a book about the hospital stayed with me; and when the war in Ukraine broke out in February 2022, I realized that under the current circumstances I needed to take the lead.

Each of the experts I contacted during the spring and summer of 2022 graciously agreed to contribute to *Visionaries from Lviv: The Story of a Jewish Hospital* and provided three remarkable chapters on the history of Jewish medicine in Galicia (especially Lviv), the fascinating architecture of the Lazarus Jewish Hospital and the people behind it, and the hospital's activities and its role in the Jewish community and city as a whole. My own chapter, a biography of Maurycy Lazarus, was much more difficult to write than I originally expected, as the more I learned about him, the more there was to discover—and I suspect there still is.

In the book, we have tried to link the history of the Jewish Hospital, and the people involved with it, to the broader history of Habsburg Galicia after the 1772 Partition of Poland between Russia, Austria, and Prussia. Those we have termed the "Visionaries from Lviv" lived at a time when the city was truly multiethnic, with more than half of the population consisting of Roman Catholics (mainly Poles), one-third Jews, and about one-fifth

Greek Catholics (mainly Ruthenians—i.e., Ukrainians). The creation of the Lazarus Jewish Hospital was a shared effort involving prestigious representatives of all three communities.

In chapter one, "Jewish Medical Practitioners from Galicia: Barber-Surgeons, Physicians, and Societal Trailblazers," Andrew Zalewski discusses the long tradition among Polish Jews to engage in medical profession and describes the impact of early Jewish physicians on opening Jewish community to the currents of modernization. He also writes about the first women doctors—who happened to be Jewish—educated in Lviv.

In chapter two, "Maurycy Lazarus, Founder of the Jewish Hospital, and His Family," I draw on both documentary evidence and family stories to place Maurycy Lazarus—both his life and work—in the context of the nineteenth- and twentieth-century history of Galicia. I further describe the roles played by Zionism and socialism at the turn of the twentieth century in his children's lives.

In chapter three, "The Jewish Hospital in Lemberg/Lwów/Lviv: Its Architecture and Architects," Sergey Kravtsov explores how the architecture of the hospital fits into the cityscape and how it was a product of the minds of a Jewish philanthropist, a Ukrainian master builder, and a Polish architect, all of them complex personalities with very different political views.

In chapter four, "The Maurycy Lazarus Foundation Israelite Hospital (1903–1939)," Anna Jakimyszyn-Gadocha describes the workings of the hospital, the most modern institution of its kind in Galicia at the time, and sketches profiles of its doctors. She details the role of the hospital in the Jewish community and the city between 1903, when it opened, and the beginning of World War II in 1939.

The contributors to *Visionaries from Lviv: The Story of a Jewish Hospital*—variously from the United States, Israel, and Poland—have tried to demonstrate the Jewish Hospital's past and present importance for Lviv. As one of the few still operational pre-Second World War Jewish institutions, now a municipal one, the hospital acts as a reminder of the once vibrant Jewish community of Lviv that was totally annihilated during the Holocaust. It also shows how one person's dream and commitment can impact the lives of many and proves that, given the opportunity, people of different religions, ethnicities, or nationalities can join to build something inspiring and permanent.

Ewa Herbst
Edgewater, New Jersey, 2024

Chapter 1

Jewish Medical Practitioners from Galicia: Barber-Surgeons, Physicians, and Societal Trailblazers[*]

Andrew Zalewski

For millennia, Jews were drawn to the art of healing by ethical considerations, interest in rational inquiry, and the desire to earn respect in society. The Hebrew word *hesed* (loving kindness) is rooted in biblical texts and implies compassionate action on behalf of someone in need which is the basic foundation of medical ethics. Several references to health, disease, and physicians are found in the Talmud. In the Middle Ages, Jewish medical practitioners achieved prominence in northern Africa and on the Iberian Peninsula under Islamic rule. The Sephardic Jews brought from Spain to the rest of Europe a "Hebrew library," the body of medical texts translated from Arabic, which were largely unknown to the Christian world. Under the influence of Jewish tradition, the desire of Jewish communities to offer shelter to strangers, to the poor, and to the sick led to the emergence of a *beth hekdesh haanim* (a house consecrated to the needy). After appearing first in thirteenth-century Ashkenazi

---

[*] I wish to thank Tony Kahane, Steven Turner, and Mark Jacobson from Gesher Galicia for their interest and helpful discussions during the Jewish medical students research project. The advice of Jay Osborn about historical maps of Galicia, some of which are featured in this chapter, invariably uncovered a number of important details. Rabbi Edward Reichman, MD, professor of emergency medicine, Albert Einstein College of Medicine, New York, and Isaac and Bella Tendler Chair in Jewish Medical Ethics, Yeshiva University, New York, generously shared with me his discoveries and sources pertaining to Jewish students at Padua University in the early modern period. My thanks also extend to Dr. László Molnár, head of the Semmelweis University Archives, Hungary, who shared with me information about many Jewish students from Galicia. I am also grateful to Dr. Agnieszka Franczyk-Cegła, head of the Early Imprints Department, Ossolineum Institute, Wrocław, Poland, who aided my research with important archival sources, including those on early Jewish surgeons.

communities in German cities, they later spread through eastern Europe, becoming precursors of the modern-era Jewish hospital.[1]

Until the end of the eighteenth century, medicine was the only field of secular science in which Jews could engage and gain positive recognition in wider society. More recent writings underscored the multidimensional role of university-trained doctors, who on occasion, transmitted nonmedical discoveries to the Jewish world.[2] From the perspective of their still largely separate communities, many Jewish physicians became the first messengers of acculturation.[3]

The history of Jews pursuing medicine as a vocation in Galicia begins before the First Partition of Poland and continues through the Austrian period (1772–1918). Transition from a Jewish practitioner previously apprenticed in just a few rudimentary skills to a university-educated physician often had a modernizing influence on the Jewish community beyond the practice of medicine. Many of those physicians, initially only men, were active in Lviv, being directly or indirectly affiliated with the Jewish hospital. Jewish women physicians joined the hospital in Lviv only at the beginning of the twentieth century. On the path to professional careers, they had to overcome different barriers than their male counterparts had generations earlier.

Before Austrian Galicia (pre-1772)

Long before the partitions of the Polish-Lithuanian Commonwealth and the emergence of Habsburg Galicia, Jewish doctors were sought for their talents by the Polish Crown. After the expulsion of Jews from Spain in 1492, a small number of Sephardic Jews arrived in Poland, where some served as court physicians. Isaac Hispanus (?–1510), previously at the court of a Persian shah, attended to the medical needs of four consecutive Polish kings. By royal decrees, Hispanus was granted rewards from the obligations paid by local Ashkenazi Jews to the Crown. He was also exempted from taxes and placed outside the Jewish traditional communal jurisdiction. This privileged status and Sephardic background created tensions between Hispanus and the Ashkenazic Jews in Kraków.

---

1 Harry Friedenwald, *The Jews and Medicine*, 2 vols. (Baltimore: Johns Hopkins Press, 1944), 1:5–30; on Judaism and healing, as well as on rabbinic laws governing the practice of medicine, 1:185–216; on Jewish medical practitioners under Islam, 1:613–700; on Jews and medicine on the Iberian Peninsula, 2:514–518; on Jewish hospitals, Domus Hospitale Judeorum in Regensburg in 1210, Cologne in 1248; Cecil Roth, "The Qualification of Jewish Physicians in the Middle Ages," *Speculum* 28, no. 4 (1953): 834–836.
2 See Isaac Barzilay, *Yoseph Shlomo Delmedigo (Yashar of Candia): His Life, Work and Times* (Leiden: E. J. Brill, 1974), 125–133, 151–166, on the physician-scientist Joseph Delmedigo (1591–1655) and the heliocentric theory in *Sefer Elim* (1629); David B. Ruderman, *Jewish Thought and Scientific Discovery in Early Modern Europe* (New Haven: Yale University Press, 1995), 115–117, on Jewish graduates from Padua University and their contacts with the non-Jewish world.
3 Majer Bałaban, on early Jewish physicians in Poland, several contributions cited in the text; John M. Efron, *Medicine and the German Jews: A History* (New Haven and London: Yale University Press, 2001), 34–40, 64–104, on Jewish doctors in German lands.

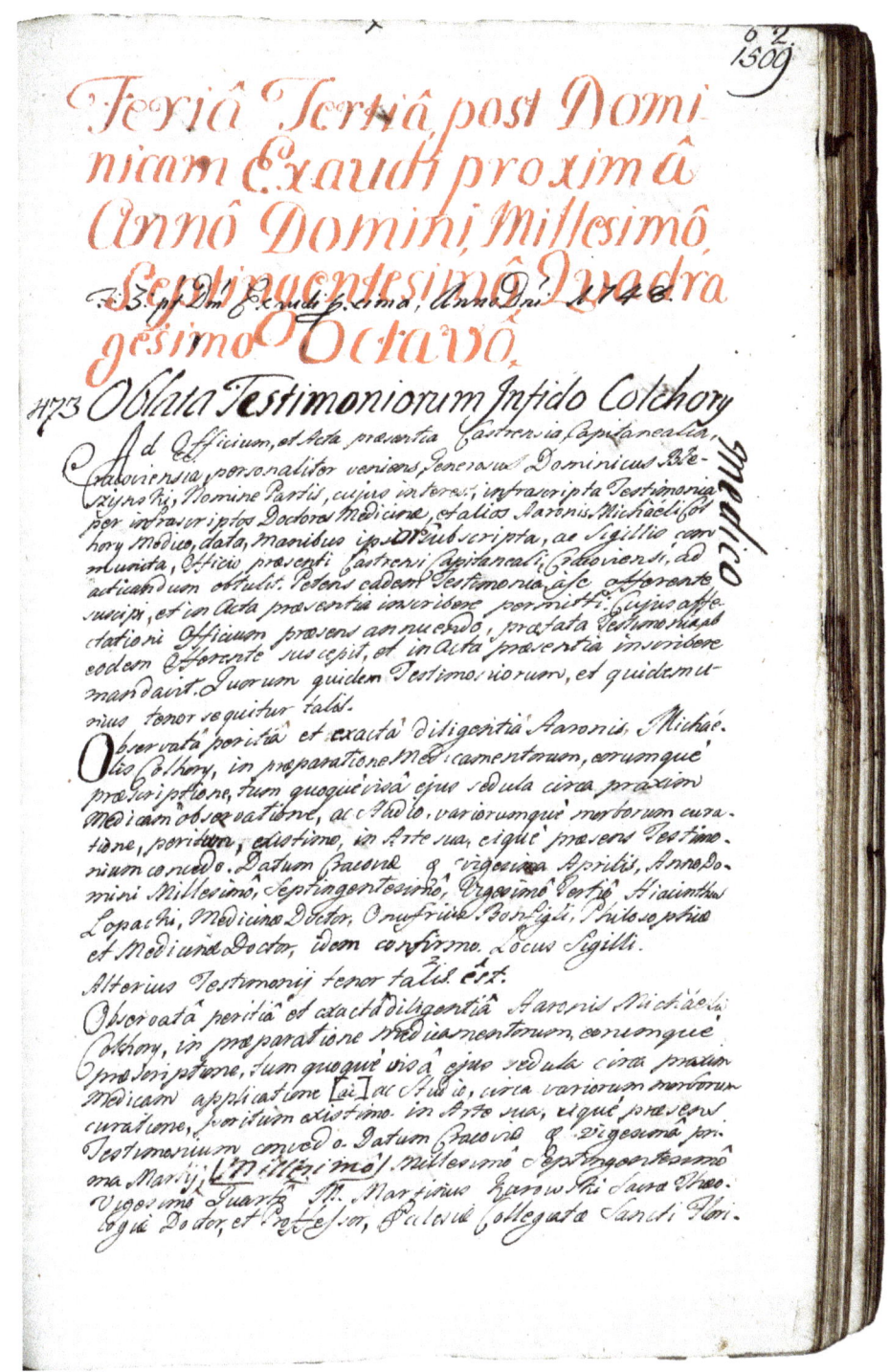

Figure 1.1. Aron Calahora (referred to as "infido Colchory medico") found qualified to practice medicine by the Jagiellonian University professors, 1723–1727. At the time, Jews were not admitted to the university in Kraków. He was a descendant of Salomon Calahora. Acta Castrensia Cracoviensa, Relationes, 1752–1796. ANK, 29/5/0/2/850, f. 1509.

The medical professionals who served the Polish Crown also included Italian Jews. The surgeon Samuel bar Meshulam was brought by Italian-born Queen Bona Sforza, who resided in Kraków. After his death, the physician Solomon Ashkenazi from Udine became the court physician before moving on to the Ottoman Empire in 1565. At that time, Salomon Kalahora (?–1597; Calahora, Colhori), a Sephardic Jew whose family had roots in the Iberian Peninsula, was already living in Kraków. He was appointed court doctor in 1570, and his descendants would continue to live in Poland for the next three centuries (fig. 1.1). Under royal patronage, Kalahora received lucrative commercial rights to the salt trade, a pricey commodity at the time.[4]

During the next two centuries, the medical profession in the Polish-Lithuanian Commonwealth continued to attract Jews, both foreign and locally born. At the same time, the role of these physicians took on a new dimension. Moving with greater ease between the Jewish and Christian worlds, prominent doctors sometimes acted as intercessors (*shtadlanim*), interfacing with the authorities on behalf of their coreligionists.[5] On other occasions, they mediated internal Jewish conflicts. Two physicians—Emanuel DeJona (d. 1702; de Jona, Simcha Menachem), and later, Abraham Isaac Fortis (d. circa 1731)—presided over the Council of Four Lands, the pan-communal Jewish assembly in the Polish-Lithuanian Commonwealth. DeJona, who was from a distinguished medical family in Lviv, was also the royal physician. He demonstrated his pan-communal leadership by successfully resolving a brewing dispute among the Hebrew printing houses. Fortis, who was born in Italy, also periodically lived in Lviv. Highly educated and fluent in Latin, he was a shrewd politician who despite his foreign roots, rapidly ascended to the leadership of the council in 1724.[6]

But for Jewish doctors, gaining prestige could easily become a double-edged sword. One particularly noxious publication denounced those who use "Jews, Tatars, and other infidels as physicians, and pass to others their advice ... or cause others to seek their services against prohibitions by the Holy Universal Church." The author, a medical doctor himself, warned that reliance on such "infidels" placed the patient's soul and body in mortal danger.[7] The accusations Christian doctors threw at Jewish medical practitioners, especially after the death of a famous patient and in cases of petty professional jealousy, could also easily lead to judicial proceedings with serious consequences. To this end, Emanuel DeJona was briefly imprisoned after his patient, King Jan Sobieski, died in 1696, and the brother of Abraham Isaac Fortis, who was also a physician, was sued in the Crown Tribunal on a ludicrous charge in 1710.[8]

---

4 Majer Bałaban, *Historja Żydów w Krakowie i na Kazimierzu 1304–1868*, 2 vols. (Kraków: Nadzieja, 1931), 1:82–83, 140–142, 151–153, and Majer Bałaban, *Z historji Żydów w Polsce* (Warszawa: Lewin-Epstein, 1920), 90–91, on foreign and local Jews.
5 Efron, *Medicine and the German Jews*, 43–44, for the contrast with Jewish doctors in Germany, where they were excluded from the communal leadership and lacked financial influence, which was exerted by Court Jews (Hofjuden).
6 Judith Kalik, "Office Holders of the Council of Four Lands, 1595–1764," in *Jewish Self-Government in Eastern Europe*, ed. François Guesnet and Antony Polonsky (London: Littman Library, 2022), 131–132; Bałaban, *Z historji Żydów w Polsce*, 49–57, on DeJona's leadership in c. 1699.
7 Sebastyan Śleszkowski, *Iasne dowody o doktorach żydowskich* (Kraków, 1649), 1–2, the book continued to be reprinted until the 1750s.
8 Bałaban, *Z historji Żydów w Polsce*, 94–97, the pharmacist Mattathias Kalahora was burned at the stake (1663); Bałaban, "Lekarze żydowscy w dawnej Rzeczypospolitej," in *Żydzi w Polsce odrodzonej*, 2 vols., ed. I. Schiper et al.

A profession in transition

Two different and competing approaches to the medical education coexisted over the centuries. The older approach was apprenticeship-based training of healers (*medicus*), which followed oral tradition and the mechanical repetition of tasks. Beginning in the Middle Ages, this system was slowly supplanted by university education, where physicians (*physicus*) or surgeons were taught in institutional settings.[9] This latter approach involved learning about the causes of disease based on the emerging science and formed the foundation of rational medicine. The first universities traced their beginnings to medieval Italy. Typically, they began as law schools (colleges of jurists), with medical schools added only later as part of the college of arts. The oldest university was established in Bologna in 1088, followed by another one in Padua in 1222.[10] During this period, other cities in Italy and in France (for example, Paris and Montpellier) also embraced this new trend of scholastic medicine.

By the fourteenth century, some Jews became drawn to the new study of medicine. One of them wrote: "I went to . . . the renowned city, to hear the science of medicine from the mouth of Christian doctors and scholars, and there I found numerous books and useful commentaries."[11] What had initially started with fleeting encounters—hearing lectures, meeting professors, and later translating medical treatises from Latin to Hebrew—would soon develop into Jews desiring a full learning experience. This aspiration, though, was most often denied by the ecclesiastical powers controlling higher education, as the Church barred Jews from gaining academic degrees.

The University of Padua was a notable exception. Soon after the Republic of Venice took control of the city, the first degree in medicine was conferred on a Jew in 1409. Even the papal bull of 1564, which mandated graduating students to profess the Catholic faith in the Sacred College, with a bishop and the university hierarchy in attendance, did not halt completing medical studies by non-Catholics. The imperial officials (Counts Palatine) could confer degrees on Protestants and Jews, thus circumventing the papal decree. In 1616, the authorities established the Venetian College of Arts (Collegio Veneto Artista) in Padua. This body of professors and other doctors was empowered to issue degrees in philosophy and medicine to "poor students and others," the latter denoting non-Catholics. In the next hundred years (1619–1721), 149 doctoral diplomas were received by Jews (fig. 1.2). Among them were three generations of the DeJona family from Lviv, a few Morpurgos from Kraków, and Gabriel Felix from Brody, as well as several Gordons from Vilna, and

---

(Warszawa, 1932), 1: 299–300; on another Fortis, see M. J. Rosman, *The Lord's Jews: Magnate-Jewish Relations in the Polish-Lithuanian Commonwealth during the 18th Century* (Cambridge, MA: Harvard University Press, 1990), 149–153, 180–181. Moses Fortis, who served as a doctor and agent (factor) for the Polish nobility, was faced with charges and fled abroad (1720s).

9 Jerome J. Bylebyl, "The Medical Meaning of Physica," *Osiris* 6, no. 1 (1990): 16, 38–40.

10 Piero Del Negro, ed. *University of Padua: Eight Centuries of History* (Padova: Signumpadova, 2003), 15–16, 153. After the law school was established, the medical school opened around 1250.

11 Luis Garcia-Ballester, Lolla Ferre, and Eduard Feliu, "Jewish Appreciation of Fourteenth-Century Scholastic Medicine," *Osiris* 6, no. 1, (1990): 93, 96, 116; the quote is by Abraham Abigdor, translator of medical books, visiting Montpellier.

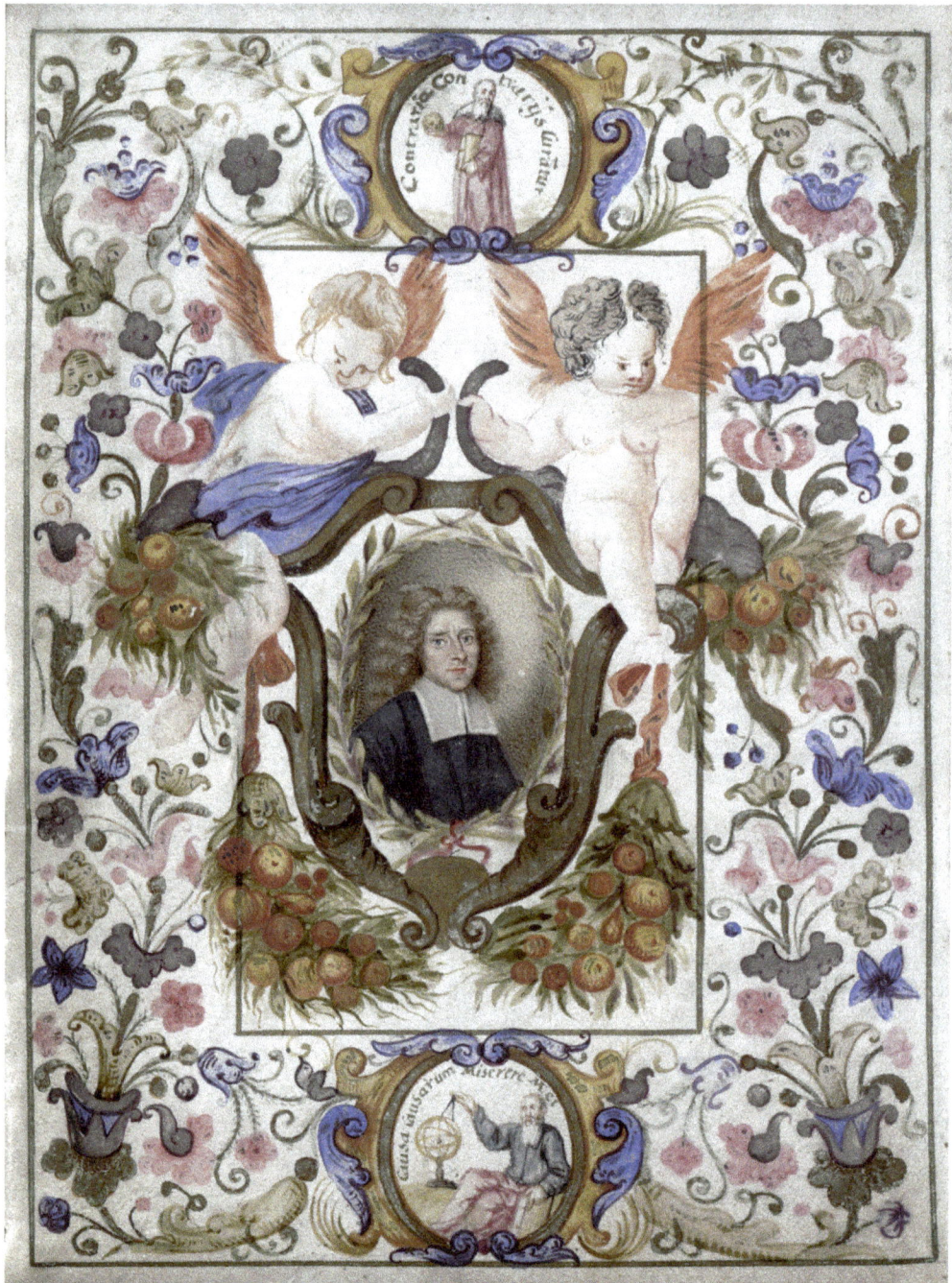

Figure 1.2. Diploma of doctor of medicine awarded to Koppel Mehler (Latinized name Copilius Pictorius) from Bingen in Germany, issued by Padua University, 1695. Above: the graduate's portrait. Opposite page: for Jewish graduates, the invocation began "In Dei Aeterni nomine . . ." (in the name of eternal God) instead of "In Christi nomine . . ." (in the name of Christ), reserved for Christians. NLI, 990034210990205171.

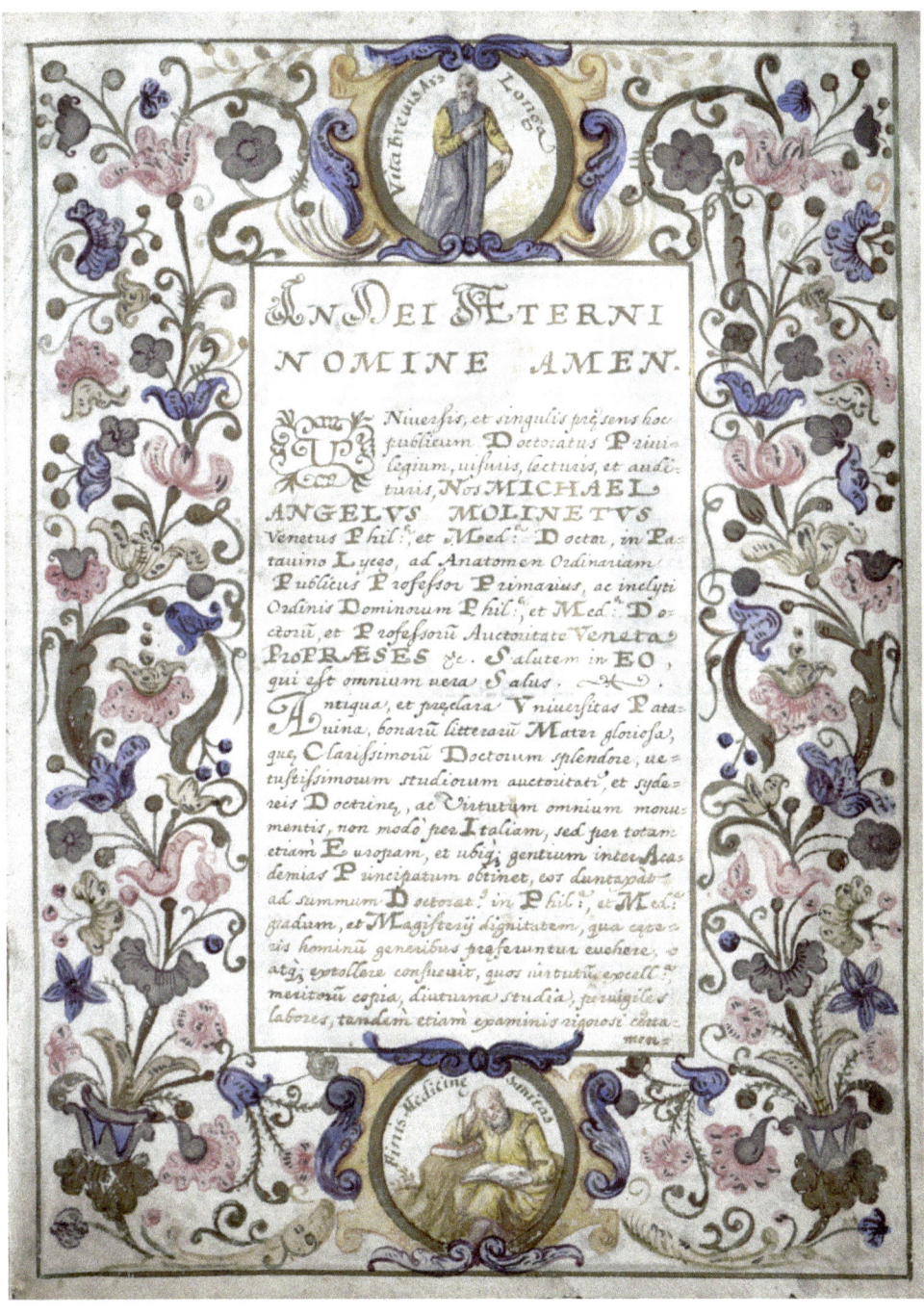

others.[12] Returning home, a lucky graduate was often referred to as a *"rofeh mumcheh* (expert physician)."[13]

After Padua and a few other Italian universities, German universities relaxed their admission policies. The university in Frankfurt an der Oder allowed Jews to study medicine in 1678, though at first without earning degrees. Writing from Halle, where another university was located, an exuberant Jewish medical student told a friend in 1702 that he was allowed to carry a sword like other students there![14] Later in the eighteenth century, the first doctoral degrees were granted to Jewish students in several German universities, including Frankfurt an der Oder (1721), Halle (1724), Heidelberg (1728), and Königsberg (1781). Frankfurt, as the city of frequent exchanges with eastern Europe, attracted the largest number of Jews from the Polish territories.[15]

The medical marketplace at home

Despite growing access to university-based medical knowledge, Jews nevertheless faced challenges arising from within their own community. Among the Ashkenazim, rabbinic authorities held a tight monopoly on Jewish education. While a number of Italian rabbis provided a supportive environment for medical students, the rabbis in pre-partition Poland remained ambivalent about the university studies outside their control. In particular, the study of philosophy was perceived as a threat to Jewish identity, which was shaped almost exclusively by ubiquitous religious education. Beyond a few exceptions, the Jews of eastern Europe lacked the role model of a rabbi-physician open to secular knowledge, as was found among Italian Jewry. There were also practical considerations: foreign schools were far away and costly, charging Jews considerably higher fees than other students. In addition, there were disadvantages related to the traditional Jewish educational system. For example, Latin, the language of instruction at the university, was not taught in a Jewish religious school (*heder*) in eastern Europe.[16]

Not surprisingly, most Jewish medical practitioners followed a less controversial and more affordable path by becoming barber-surgeons (in Polish, *cyrulik* or *balwierz*; in

---

12 Friedenwald, *The Jews and Medicine*, 1:225–227, 253–256; by comparison, eighty Jews received doctoral degrees in 1517–1619; Jan Warchał, "Żydzi polscy na uniwersytecie padewskim," *Kwartalnik Żydów w Polsce* 1, no. 3 (1913): 37–72, the university archive excerpts; Del Negro, *University of Padua*, 51–53, on granting degrees; on Gabriel Felix from Galicia, see Edward Reichman, "Notes on the Jewish Renaissance Physician Gabriel Felix: His Grammar Tree and His Family Tree," *Korot* 25 (2019–2020): 339–353.
13 Isak N. Gath, "The Elusive Karaite Doctor Joseph Ezra Dubitski," *Karaite Archives* 3, no. 1 (2015): 27, on different appellations among medical practitioners.
14 Friedenwald, *The Jews and Medicine*, 1:237, on Isaac Wallich's letter.
15 Monika Richarz, *German Jews and the University, 1678–1848* (Rochester: Camden House, 2022), 44–46, 50, 59; Jews were admitted without the right to practice medicine there; only one-third of registered Jewish students continued to the doctorate.
16 Jacob Shatzky, "On Jewish Medical Students of Padua," *Journal of the History of Medicine and Allied Sciences* 5, no. Autumn (1950): 446, on fees paid in Padua; Richarz, *German Jews*, 48—in 1750, Jews paid twice as much in Frankfurt an der Oder and Königsberg; Ruderman, *Jewish Thought and Scientific Discovery*, 112, 256–259, on Italian rabbi-physicians, Solomon Conegliano from Padua, Isaac Lampronti from Ferrara, Joseph Cases of Siena; and 101–102, 118–120, on Leon of Modena.

German, *Balbiere* or *Bader*). In the royal towns, they belonged to a local guild of barbers, typically separate from the Christian guild, which oversaw the apprenticeships, controlled membership, and collected accompanying fees. The guild also guarded against nonmembers attempting to practice surgery in the town. In this competitive environment, a Christian guild sometimes invoked its own royal privileges that had placed limits on a number of Jewish barber-surgeons permitted to practice, as was the case in Lviv. By contrast, in the private towns owned—or received through royal patronage—by the nobility, the guilds had fewer powers or were nonexistent.[17] Thus, even though apprentices were to train for a minimum of three years, the qualifications of many barber-surgeons across the country remained uncertain at best. In the busy medical marketplace of the eighteenth-century Polish-Lithuanian Commonwealth, one could also find itinerant kabbalistic healers (*ba'alei shem*), who blended Jewish mysticism and herbal remedies with tidbits of informally acquired medical experience.[18]

Austrian Galicia (1772–1918)

"Everyone could claim to be a physician in Poland," lamented Dr. Franciscus de Luz from Naples, who happened to be in Lviv when the Austrians arrived in the fall of 1772. "I watched this with pain," he continued, "but if I said something I was guilty of treason taking away their freedoms. The Jews here practice medicine and surgery; and good midwives are rare."[19] When early the next year, two physicians and three surgeons—all recently educated at Vienna University—arrived in Lviv, their mission to organize medical services appeared to be a daunting task (fig. 1.3).[20]

In past years, the institutions of higher learning in Lviv, Zamość, and Kraków (the latter being just outside the newly established border) had either stopped granting medical degrees due to the lack of qualified professors or were prevented from doing so by conflicts among the schools. In all of Galicia—a province of more than two million people—only a handful of qualified physicians were found, and there was not a single midwife with proper training. In Lviv, a city of approximately twenty thousand, there were six non-Jewish physicians, of whom only two (both French doctors) were able to show their medical credentials.

---

17 Mark Wischnitzer, *A History of Jewish Crafts and Guilds* (New York: Davide Publishers, 1965), 210–216, 250; the Jewish guild of barbers in Kraków had its statues since 1639.
18 Yohanan Petrovsky-Shtern, "The Master of an Evil Name: Hillel Ba'al Shem and his Sefer ha-heshek," *AJS Review* 28, no. 2 (2004): 221–226, 242, 246–247; Hillel Ba'al Shem was an expert in Kabbalah and had contacts with renowned Jewish doctors in the 1730s.
19 Władysław Szumowski, *Galicja pod względem medycznym za Jędrzeja Krupińskiego pierwszego protomedyka 1772–1783* (Lwów: Towarzystwo Popierania Nauki Polskiej, 1907), 34, 302; see also Andrew Zalewski, "Becoming Habsburg Galitzianers," *Galitzianer* 26, no. 3 (2019): 12–17, on the First Partition of Poland, and "The First Habsburg Census"; *Galitzianer* 26, no. 4 (2019): 6–10, on population statistics and conditions in 1773.
20 "Statuit Provinciales Medicos," in *Edicta et Mandata Universalia Regnis Galiciae et Lodomeriae* (Lwów: J. Piller, 1773), 45–50; Jędrzej Krupiński and Johann Spaventi were appointed to oversee medical affairs in Galicia—they were assisted by Johann Waltz, Franz Ogesser, and Anton Kremler (March 20, 1773).

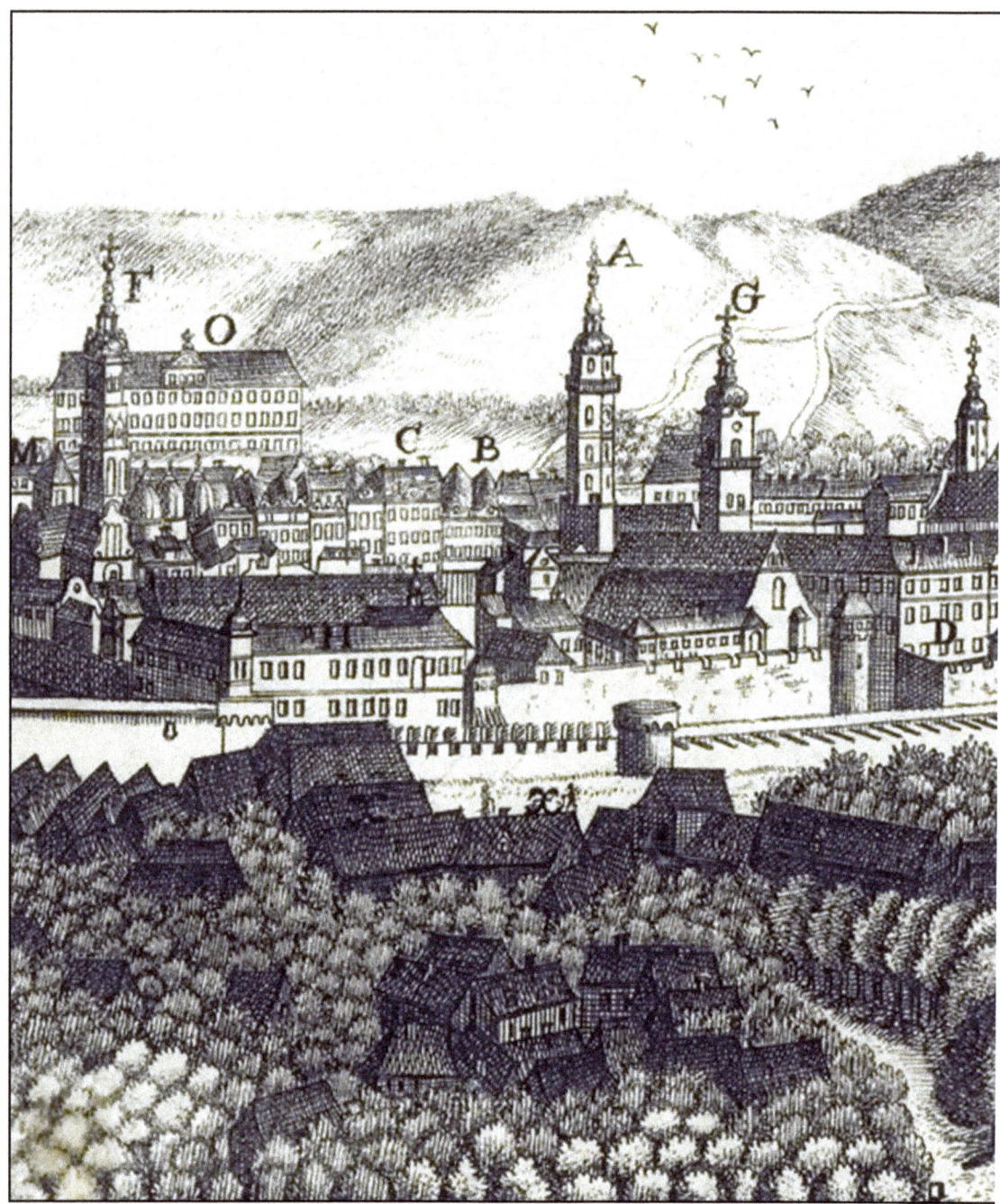

Figure 1.3. The capital city of Lviv in the 1770s. In the foreground (opposite page), the Jewish cemetery marked by headstones (R) and Jewish dwellings in the outer Kraków suburb (Krakauer Vorstadt), the location of the future Jewish hospital. In the background (both pages), the inner city, with the city hall (A), the governor's residence (B), the military garrison (C), and the towers of several churches (D–G). The city was surrounded by walls and a moat (L). A section of the engraving by François Perneuer. POLONA, G.27995.

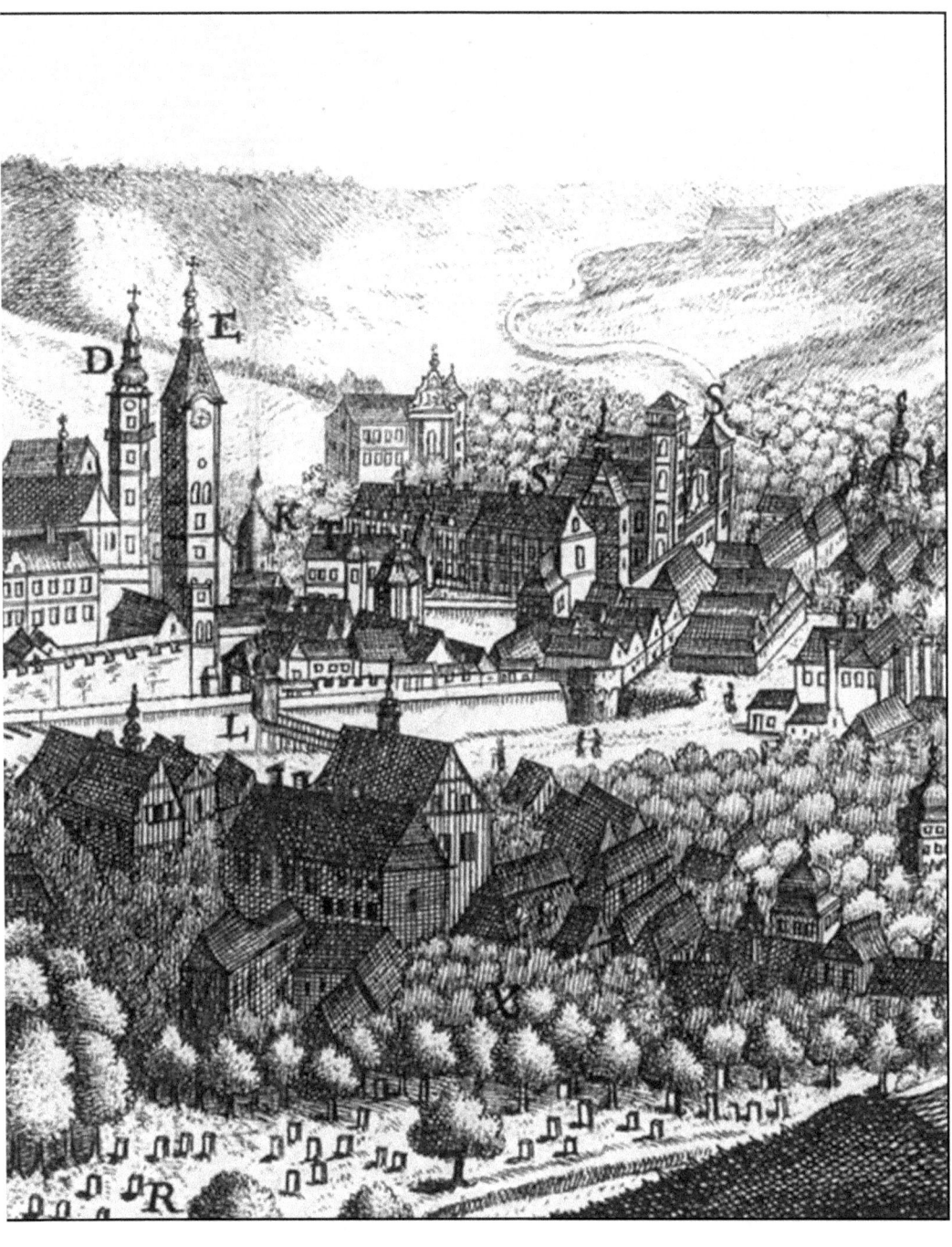

The others claimed to have been educated elsewhere in Europe, though the proof was hard to come by. Outside the capital city of Galicia, a few qualified Jewish physicians were identified by the new medical authorities. Moses Lewin in Zamość had graduated from Frankfurt University. Abraham Uziel in Brody had also studied in German lands. Fluent in several languages, he served as a spokesman for the Jewish community. Samuel Rosenberg, another physician living in Brody, had completed with distinction medical courses at the universities in The Hague and in Frankfurt an der Oder, though he was unable to present his medical diploma.[21]

Rosenberg was originally from Vienna, the home of a newly reformed university, with a first-class academic medical faculty, which incorporated into its curriculum the practice of bedside teaching—quite revolutionary for the times. The engine behind these sweeping changes was a Dutch physician, Gerhard van Swieten, who had made Vienna University one of the best universities in Europe. Van Swieten was respected by Maria Theresa, the sovereign of the Austrian Monarchy, serving not only as her court physician, but also as the head of academic reforms and public health policies.[22]

Unfortunately, Van Swieten threw his weight behind the ban of non-Catholics from the University of Vienna. Even medical degrees earned abroad could not guarantee them professional recognition. As late as 1771, the "great Van Swieten"—as Maria Theresa referred to her doctor—issued a rebuke of Prague University on hearing that Jews educated elsewhere were credentialed there. "I believe that the same law applies to Bohemia," he wrote with scorn. "If we would observe the law, they would never admit Jews to the examinations.... Never, a Jew is allowed to be examined in Vienna; we always refuse for these reasons."[23] In this climate, Jewish doctors back in Galicia were sometimes suspected of fraud when they presented foreign diploma to a provincial chief medical administrator (*Protomedicus*) in charge of medical licensing.

With so few physicians, a number of Jewish barber-surgeons practiced throughout Galicia, with nineteen of them in Lviv alone.[24] Those authorized by the guild displayed signs with a washbasin in front of their establishments. Besides cutting hair, they performed bloodletting, practiced rudimentary dentistry, treated external wounds, and applied fire cupping. The barber-surgeons were also trained in bandaging hernias and setting bone fractures. Among the Jewish barber-surgeons, only one was formally trained; others presented patient testimonies attesting to their success in medical procedures. Less than a year after the Austrian control of Galicia was established, barber-surgeons were forbidden to treat internal ailments, unless there was no qualified physician in the area.[25]

---

21 Szumowski, *Galicia pod względem medycznym*, 28, 50–53, 70; on Uziel, see Nathan Koren, *Jewish Physicians: A Biographical Index* (Jerusalem: Israel Universities Press, 1973), 133, and "Schreiben eines freundes an seinen freund von Brody in Pohlen," *Wienerisches Diarum*, January 29, 1774, unnumbered pages, the report from Brody.
22 Horace Marshall Korns, "Notes on the Medical History of Vienna," *Annals of Medical History* 9, no. 4 (1937): 350–358, on Vienna University and reforms instituted by Van Swieten.
23 Gerson Wolf, *Studies zur Jubelfeier der Wiener Univesität im Jahre 1865* (Vienna: Herzfeld & Bauer, 1865), 81–86, on Van Swieten and Jews.
24 Szumowski, *Galicia pod względem medycznym*, 54–59, 70, the information for 1773.
25 "Statuit Provinciales Medicos," in *Edicta et Mandata*, 46, 48.

Starting in 1773, free medical training was launched in Lviv twice a week in Polish and German. The lectures were open to physicians, barber-surgeons, and midwives to provide badly needed qualifications.[26] After attending three years of training and passing an examination, a graduate received a diploma. Attendance was rather poor except for one group: Lviv's Jewish barber-surgeons "were first who followed the order," read the report. "They bought books, listened attentively to lectures, a few of them even took additional private lessons; they showed fitness [to practice] during exams, and were certified as surgeons."[27]

These comments notwithstanding, the new regulations of 1776 tried to separate Jews from the rest of society, even patient care was not exempt from the anachronistic directives. Jewish doctors could "freely" practice medicine but only among other Jews. Eleven recent graduates of the medical training in Lviv appointed as regional Jewish surgeons were subordinated to a Christian physician in each district (fig. 1.4). Accredited midwives, if they happened to be Jewish, were forbidden to offer their services in Christian homes. Jewish barber-surgeons were even forbidden to shave or treat non-Jews. Those working in Lviv were warned that only four of them might be allowed to remain in the city, with the threat of expulsion hanging over them until the 1780s.[28]

The beginning of change

In 1780, Emperor Joseph II, son of Maria Theresa, became the sole ruler of the Austrian Monarchy and momentum quickly built toward enlightened reforms. Two years later, the universities in Vienna and elsewhere in the Habsburg realm opened their admissions to Jews, with the exception of the theology departments.[29] When in July 1784, the dean of the Vienna University Faculty of Medicine attempted to interfere with a Jewish physician in Prague, the Court Chancellery issued a swift response: "The professor and the medical faculty are to understand that in the future not only [Dr. Jonas] Jeiteles, but also other Jews who passed examinations and were qualified by the university are free to practice unrestricted." Joseph II also added his disapproval: "When facts are found true, Prof. Mikan must be sharply rebuked by the Gubernio."[30]

---

26 "Gratis erigitur studium artis Medicae," in *Continuatio Edictorum et Mandatorum Universalium in Regnis Galiciae et Lodomeriae* (Lwów: A. Piller, 1774), 9–10.
27 Szumowski, *Galicia pod względem medycznym*, 84–87, 331, from the report of the collegium medicum; Jews attended training given by Johann Waltz in German.
28 "Die Einführung der neuen Juden-Ordnung betreffend," in *Continuatio Edictorum* (Lwów: A. Piller, 1776), 76–121; for English translation, see Andrew Zalewski, *Galician Portraits: In Search of Jewish Roots* (Jenkintown: Thelzo Press, 2014)—see 286–341 on the legal status of the Jews; Szumowski, *Galicia pod względem medycznym*, 151–152, 165, on restrictions imposed by the Austro-Bohemian Chancellery; 163–164, on barber-surgeons in Lviv.
29 Max Neuburger, "Die ersten an der Wiener medizinischen Fakultät promovierten Arzte jüdischen Stammes," *Monatsschrift für Geschichte und Wissenschaft des Judentums* 26, no. 3 (1918): 220–221, the decree admitting Jews to Vienna University was read to professors of law and medicine on March 23, 1782, Abraham Samuel Ackord from Austria was the first Jew to graduate as a physician in Vienna in 1789.
30 Wolf, *Studies zur Jubelfeier der Wiener Universität*, 86–88, on the Gottfried Mikan affair. "Gubernio" denoted the highest office in the province.

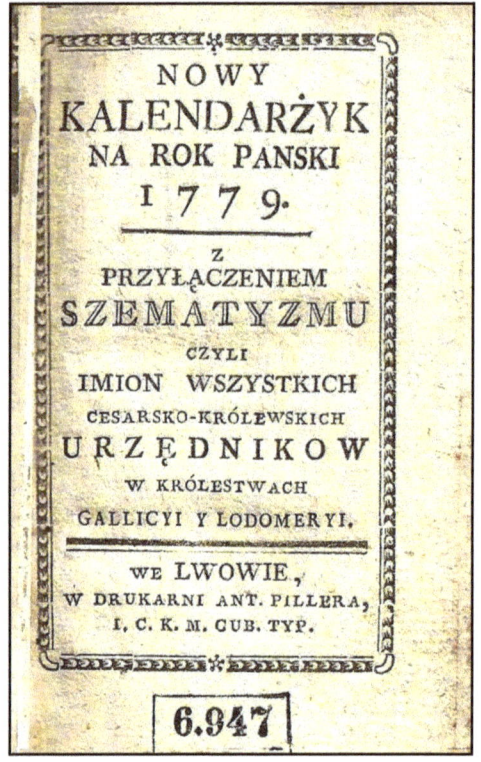
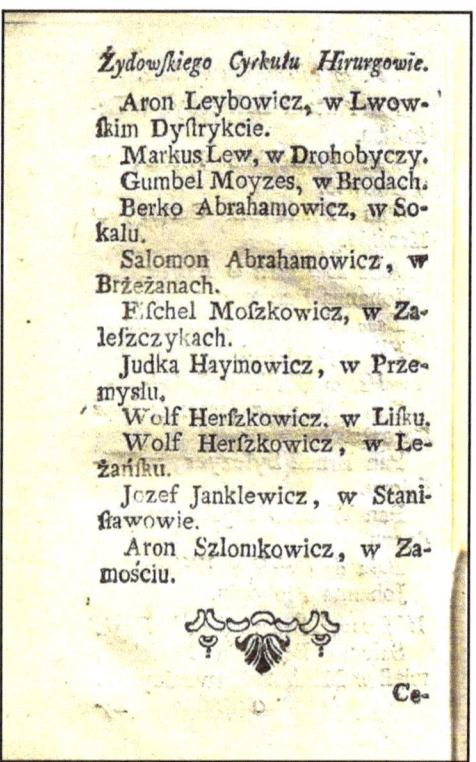

Figure 1.4. Jewish surgeons in Galicia. Left: cover page of the 1779 calendar with the listing of the Habsburg provincial bureaucracy. Right: inside page, Jewish district surgeons' names recorded in patronymic format; Jews adopted hereditary surnames only in 1788. LNNBU, CT-I 35540.

In 1784, the regulation that kept medical care separate for Jews and Christians was rescinded. As now stipulated by the authorities in Lviv, "duly certified Jews can carry out medical art and practice" and "should not be restricted in their rights of surgical practice." That same year, Salomon Benjamin Fröschel, who had lived in Lviv since 1775, was appointed district physician and would oversee the health matters of everyone regardless of religion (fig. 1.5).[31]

To direct more money to fund primary-level education, Joseph II insisted on reducing the number of universities in the Austrian Monarchy, but he made an exception for Galicia, where Lviv University opened in 1784. Medical students had a choice of two academic degrees, either that of a doctor or a magister-surgeon. Those aspiring to become doctors studied for four years (and soon for five years), with most lectures given in Latin, while the program for magister-surgeons was shorter. Lower-level surgical studies that did *not* lead to an academic degree were also introduced. This more practical track was short, initially

---

31 Szumowski, *Galicia pod względem medycznym*, 114, 166, and 335, for "Decret an das galliz. Gubernium" of September 16 and October 16, 1784." Guido Kisch, *Die Prager Universität und die Juden 1348–1848* (Amsterdam: Verlag B. R. Grüner, 1969), 44–45, 174, on Salomon Benjamin Fröschel and Prague University in 1773.

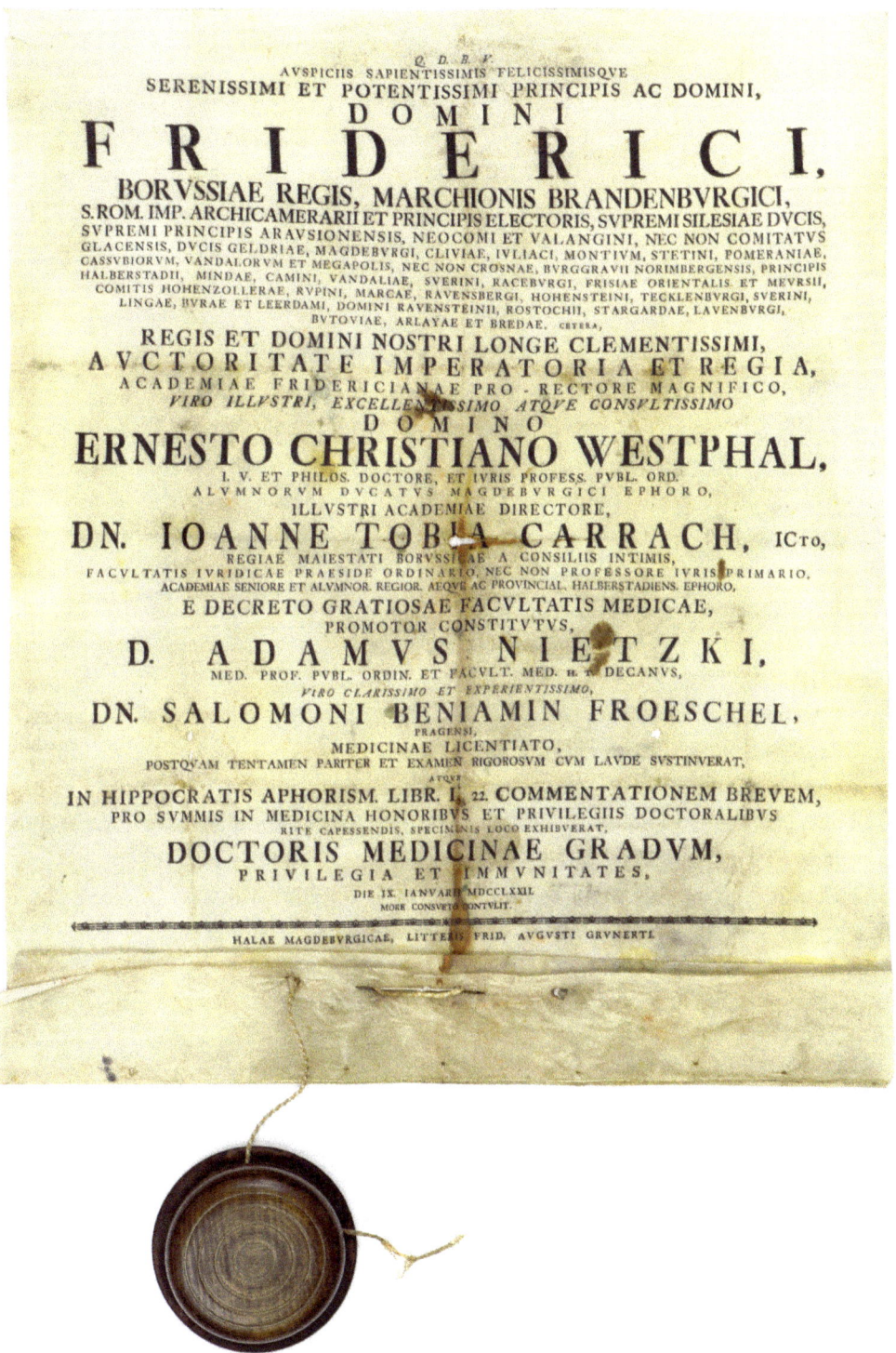

Figure 1.5. Diploma of doctor of medicine awarded to Salomon Benjamin Fröschel by Halle University, 1772. Fröschel practiced medicine in Lviv beginning in 1775, and later in Zolochiv (Złoczów). The Jewish Museum Berlin.

spread over two years, in part because Joseph II wanted to quickly train civilian surgeons (Civil- und Land-Wundärzte).[32]

Initially, the higher-level medical and surgical studies were not commonly pursued at Lviv University, with fewer than ten students found in those early years. Granting degrees was freed from religious symbolism and was conducted in the ceremony (*sponsio solemnis*) administered by the secular academic authorities. As early as 1786, the first Jewish graduate, whose name is unknown, was mentioned in passing by a visitor to Lviv.[33]

But progress was not without incident. A small group of Jews attending Lviv University was frequently harassed by their classmates on account of their appearance. After one Jewish student was physically assaulted, the authorities ordered all Jews to wear Christian-style garb to be admitted to lectures. Jewish medical students also faced burdensome residential restrictions, forcing them out of the nearby area, which was designated for Christians. Nevertheless, the number of Jews graduating from the university slowly kept rising. Soon, Christian surgeons from a few smaller towns felt threatened by the new competition. Feeling "pushed aside," as they reported "with tears," they petitioned the school to implement additional entry criteria directed exclusively at Jews. This time, the Habsburg administration in Galicia intervened and promptly rejected this demand.[34]

Other setbacks equally affected all students at the new university. A dismissal of conflict-prone professors led to a three-year suspension of medical studies beginning in 1788. Then in 1805, Lviv University was downgraded to the level of a secondary school—Lemberger Lyceum. Even though courses in surgery and midwifery were to continue, academic degrees were no longer issued by the school. To earn university-level qualifications in medicine, students had to pursue their education elsewhere.[35]

Initially, Jagiellonian University in Kraków, which had become part of Austrian Galicia (fig. 1.6) in 1796, was thought to be the place that would fill the gap. The university graduated the first Jewish surgeon, Salomon Wolf, in 1803. But with the unfolding political changes, Kraków was soon situated outside the Austrian borders again (1809–1846). During this period, relatively few Jewish students managed to graduate at Jagiellonian. In contrast with other schools, no Jews received doctoral degrees in medicine in Kraków until 1843, when Józef Oettinger (1818–1895) and Jonatan Warschauer (1820–1888)

---

32 "Betreffend die Praxis der Wundärzte," *Reichsgesetzblatt für die im Reichsrathe vertretenen Königreiche und Länder*, no. 25 (February 17, 1873): 125; the two-tier system of medical degrees was abolished in 1873. Afterwards, university medical education in Austria-Hungary led to the single degree of doctor of general medicine (Doktor der gesamten Heilkunde).
33 Franz Kratter, *Briefe über den itzigen Zustand von Galizien*, 3 vols. (Leipzig: G. Ph. Wucherers, 1786), 2:57; after a two-year course of study, it was most likely the lower-level licensure of a surgeon.
34 DALO, fond 26, op. 4, spr. 211, f. 147, Maria Horodyska, "Wydział Filozoficzny w Uniwersytecie Józefińskim, 1784–1804" (doctoral diss., Lviv University, 1933); DALO, fond 26, op. 22, spr. 2348, f. 1–3, Lviv University, on residential restrictions concerning Wolf Barth and Moses Arzt; and f. 8–10, on the petition against Jewish surgeons (1808).
35 Johann Kempel-Kürsinger, *Handbuch der Gesetzkunde*, 4 vols. (Vienna: k. k. Hof- und Staats-Aerarial Druckerei, 1830), 3:197–199. Five-year university education was required toward doctoral degrees in medicine or surgery; lower-level surgical studies lasted for two to three years (the regulations of 1804).

completed higher-level studies there.³⁶ Thus, the Habsburg universities in Vienna and Pest (Budapest, Hungary) provided more educational opportunities than Kraków, especially for the Jews of eastern Galicia.

Jewish physicians and the Haskalah

Many Jewish physicians became the embodiment of the Haskalah (the Jewish Enlightenment), which had its roots in eighteenth-century Germany. The movement sought to reform Jews through secular knowledge and the abandonment of Yiddish, the vernacular of eastern European Jewry. The aim was to create a cultured and morally improved individual. This process of self-improvement (*Bildung*) and the accompanying acculturation were viewed by the advocates of the Haskalah (maskilim) as a path leading Jews to civil and political emancipation. In the context of Galicia, the upwardly mobile maskilim railed against the rabbinic control of their communities, especially in the sphere of traditional Jewish education and cultural norms. They also vehemently opposed Hasidism.

Lviv became one of the main centers of the Galician Haskalah.³⁷ Several physicians who were members of the movement were affiliated with the Jewish hospital in Lviv. Their medical studies took them to Lviv University (Jacob Rappaport), Vienna University (Isaac Epstein, Adam Barach), and Pest University (Moritz Rappaport). In Galicia, they assumed leadership positions on the Jewish Community Council and rose to prominence in society as a whole. Their influence through a wide spectrum of nonmedical activism is particularly noteworthy.

Jacob Rappaport: Breaking barriers

Jacob Rappaport (1775–1855) was born in Uman (Humań), which at the time was still under nominal Polish sovereignty. With the area rocked by unrest, his family sought safety in neighboring Austrian Galicia when he was a child. Jacob's father, Mordechai, was a rabbi and a medical practitioner, who authored *Pleasant Words*, a discourse between a teacher and his students in Yiddish. An addendum to the book, under the title *Medicines for Children*, was reported to contain medicinal prescriptions written in Latin. Though where the older Rappaport received his education remains unclear. In 1781, he was credentialed "to heal

---

36 AUJ, S I/505, f. 31, Album C. R. Universitatis Cracoviensis, 1802–1837, and WL I/91, Akta magistrów chirurgii i położnictwa, 1798–1849, pages not numbered, for Salomon Wolf; AUJ, WL I/84 and I/86, Akta doktorantów, for Józef Oettinger and Jonatan Warschauer, respectively. Overall, sixty-three Jews studied medicine at Jagiellonian University, mainly toward lower degrees between 1801 and 1850.

37 Other places included Ternopil (Tarnopol), where Joseph Perl opened a model primary school (1813); Brody, where the Jewish community funded a secondary-level school (1818), and where Isaac Erter, a surgeon and Haskalah writer, settled; and Kraków, where Józef Oettinger, physician and head of Jewish hospital, was active in municipal politics.

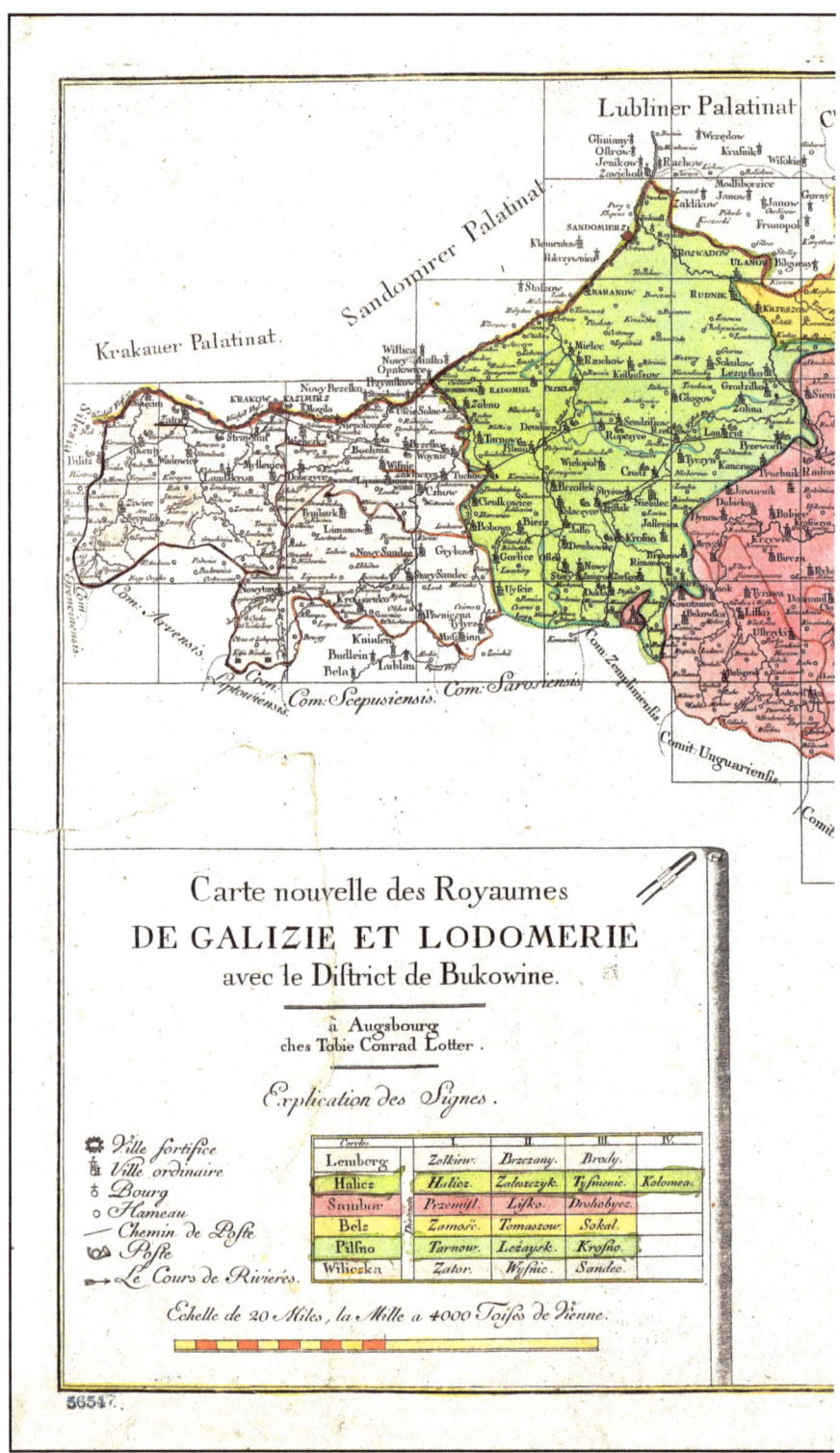

Figure 1.6. Kingdom of Galicia and Lodomeria (Königreich Galizien und Lodomerien), the official name of Austrian Galicia, c. 1780; the borders underwent adjustments in 1795, after 1809–1815 and in 1846, with Galicia remaining part of the Habsburg Empire until 1918. NYPL Digital Collections.

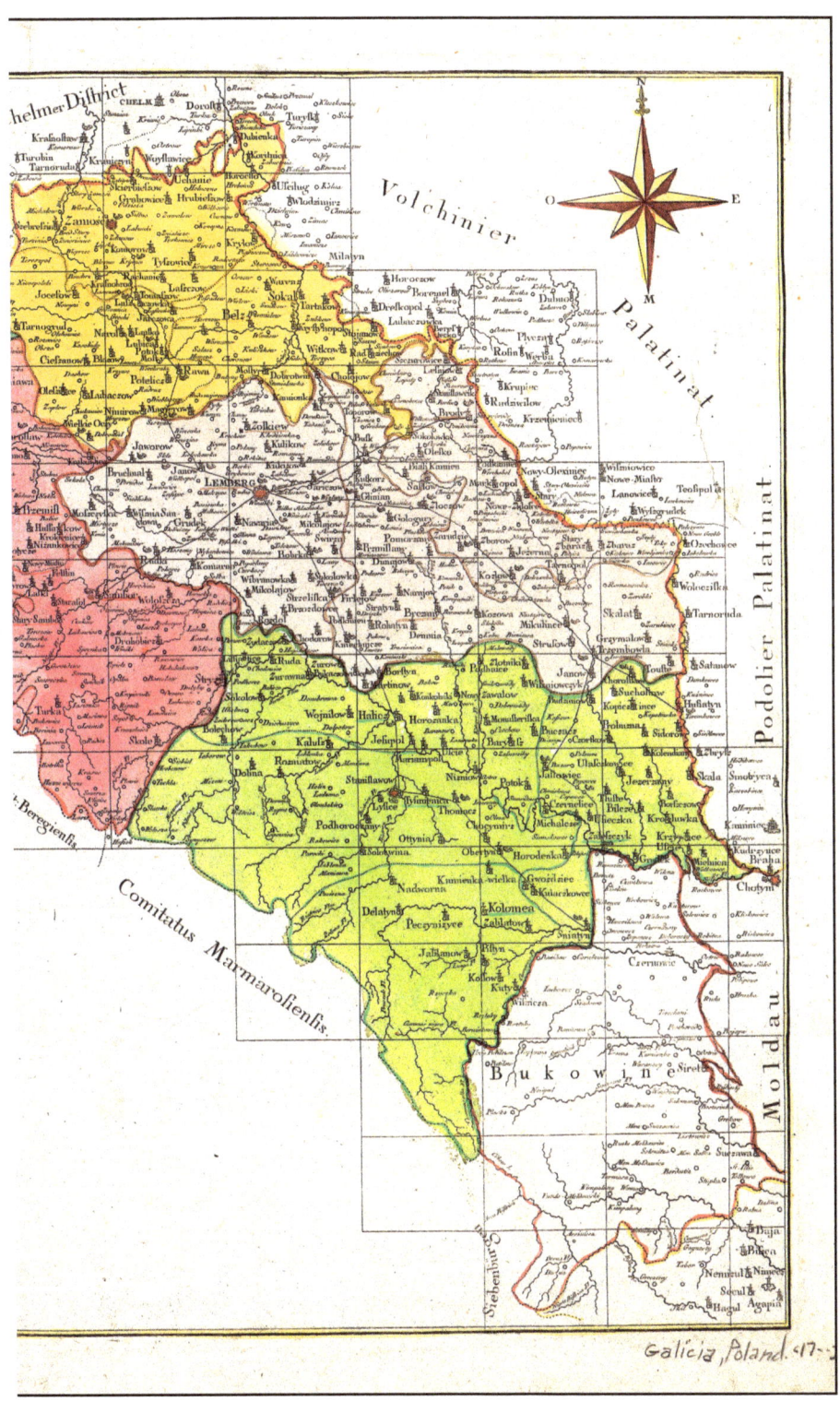

externally and internally in the entire Galicia," spent some time in Kraków, and his family would ultimately move to Stryi (Stryj), in eastern Galicia.[38]

Jacob was apparently a quick study, mastering three languages (German, Latin, and Polish) within two years. By 1798, he had already studied philosophy at Lviv University, which at the time was a prerequisite before continuing to medicine or law. University records hint at Rappaport's unique cultural exposure—he was the only Jewish student that year among his classmates, who came not only from Galicia, but also from Bohemia, Hungary, Russia, and the German states.[39] During the medical studies that followed, Rappaport was mentored by a Vienna-born professor at the university. In 1804, he became the first Jew to earn the academic degree of doctor of medicine from Lviv University (fig. 1.7).

Rappaport's medical practice transcended ethnic, religious, and economic boundaries. Early in his career, he provided free medical care to the poor when typhus spread through the city in 1806. That same year, his work at the military hospital also brought praise. At other times, he appealed in Hebrew and German to his coreligionists, combating prevalent misconceptions about the smallpox vaccination.[40]

The 1831 cholera epidemic was another event, which brought into focus Rappaport's efforts. The disease spread from Russia to Galicia, and it was rapidly moving westward through the rest of Europe. Its impact was particularly devastating in Lviv, where in the first eight months of the year about five thousand people fell ill and more than half of them died.[41] In the midst of the crisis, a visiting German physician described Rappaport as "one of the most respected Galician physicians." Recognizing his experience with the disease, he introduced Rappaport's report on cholera to German-speaking Europe when it was quickly published in Berlin. The Jewish physician from Lviv wrote of the human toll caused by cholera since time immemorial. As he put it, "people knew that the slightest contact with the sick or with his personal effects could result in illness" and "only a vile greed, the crudest ignorance . . . or high virtue and philanthropy" could overcome their fear. Working in poor neighborhoods among the sick and monitoring patients at Saint Magdalene Hospital (fig. 1.8), where a special hospital was set up (see table on page 37), Rappaport made an observation that could have saved countless lives. As he noted, "washing with a lye soap" and frequently changing clothes seemingly protected him from the disease.[42]

---

38 Majer Bałaban, *Historia lwowskiej synagogi postępowej* (Lwów: Zarząd Synagogi Postępowej, 1937), 15–16, for Mordechai Rappaport's writings; *Historja Żydów w Krakowie*, 2:537–538, 796, the license indicated "a Ukrainian rabbi, a doctor of botany and chemistry, having learned medicine . . . ," was examined in Lviv, 18 April 1781.
39 DALO, fond 26, op. 15, spr. 683, f. 372, Lviv University, Classes Auditorum Philosophiae, 1784–1815. Two to three years of study at the philosophy department were required.
40 Franz Gräffer, "Rappaport, Jacob," in *Jüdischer Plutarch*, 2 vols. (Vienna: Ulrich Klopf, 1848), 1:174–178.
41 K. B. Bicker, "Die Verbreitung der Cholera morbus im Jahre 1831," *Hesperus* 1, no. 6–7, (1832): 27; in the entire Galicia, 259,969 people contracted cholera and 97,739 of them died.
42 Jacob Rappaport, "Ueber die Contagiosität der Cholera im Vergleiche zur Pest," *Archiv für medizinische Erfahrung im Gebiete der praktischen Medizin, Chirurgie, Geburtshülfe und Staatsarzneikunde* 25 (September–October 1831): 874–876.

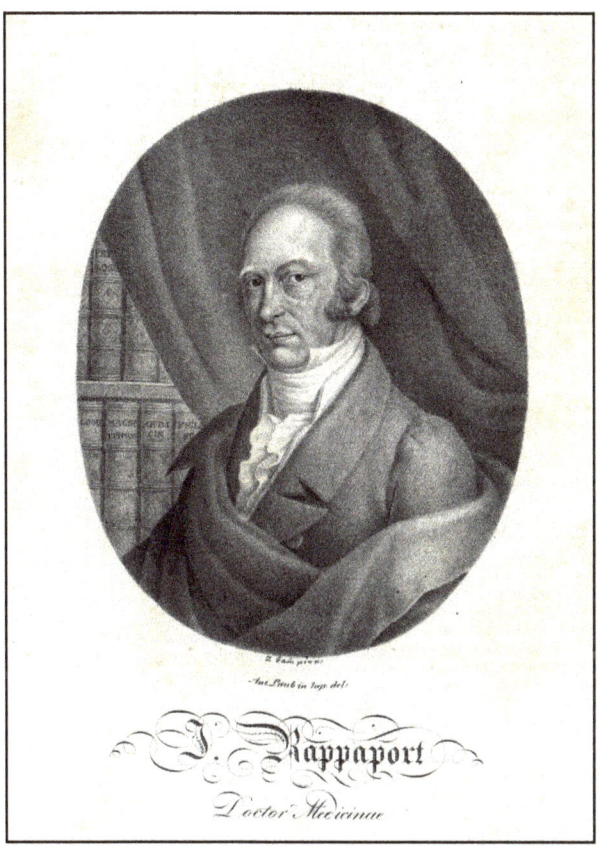

Figure 1.7. An official portrait of Jacob Rappaport, 1826. POLONA, G.10406/III.

In 1840, Jacob Rappaport was one of fifty-three Jews wanting to establish a new synagogue. Far from being a militant maskil, he sounded a cautionary note, encouraging the group to move forward with sensitivity toward the majority of Jews who did not embrace a departure from traditions of spoken language, dress code, or type of worship.

It was later said that Rappaport's signature at the top of the founding document, which included endorsements from sixteen physicians (including existing and future medical leaders of the Jewish hospital), made these delicate efforts progress more smoothly. The elegant temple, which was initially known as the German-Israelite Prayer House, and later renamed as the Progressive Synagogue, opened with fanfare in 1846.[43]

---

43 Bałaban, *Historia lwowskiej synagogi*, xvi, 17–20; Sergey R. Kravtsov, "The Progressive Synagogue in Lemberg/Lwów/Lviv," in *Jews and Slavs*, 27 vols., ed. Wolf Moskovich, Roman Mnich, and Renata Tarasiuk (Jerusalem-Siedlce: The Hebrew University of Jerusalem and Siedlce University of Natural Sciences and Humanities, 2013), 23:185–214.

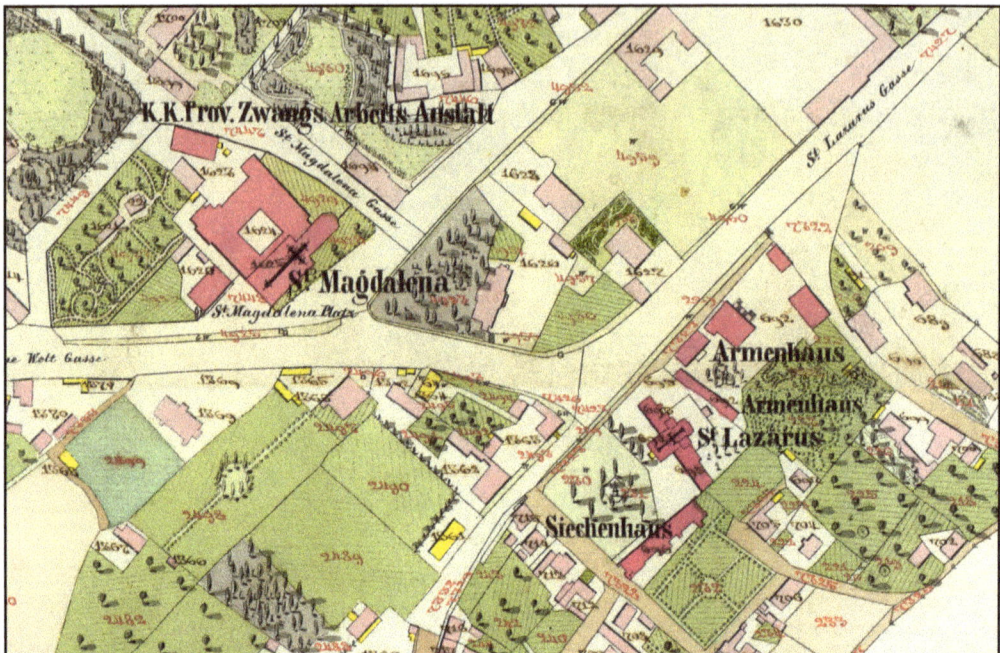

Figure 1.8. St. Magdalene and St. Lazarus hospitals in Lviv. In 1831, the building complex of St. Magdalene church served as cholera hospital (for details, see the table). A section of cadastral map of Lviv, 1849/1853. TsDIAL, fond 186, op. 8, spr. 628a.

Rappaport's life defied negative stereotypes about the Jews of Galicia. He became a corresponding member of the Society of Physicians in Vienna (k. k. Gesellschaft der Ärzte) at the organization's inception in 1837–1838.[44] Later, in 1851, after Emperor Franz Joseph established the Golden Cross, a civil decoration recognizing individuals for years of public service or other merits earned for the general good, Rappaport became an early recipient.[45]

Some years after Rappaport's death, he was memorialized when the street next to the Jewish hospital was named in his honor. The city's character kept changing, reflecting larger historical events—its name reverting from German Lemberg to Polish Lwów, and then becoming Soviet Lvov. In this kaleidoscope of cultural, political, and linguistic twists and turns, the name Rappaport Street remained constant from the early 1870s to 1941. And then, after the hiatus of the postwar Soviet period, the original street name was restored in 2011, in what is Ukrainian Lviv.[46]

---

44 In December 1837, the nominations were submitted by chief medical administrators (Protomediker) in each province of the Austrian Empire. Rappaport's name was among the first group of the members from outside Vienna.

45 "Oesterreichischer Kaiserstaat," *Allgemeine Zeitung des Judenthums*, November 24, 1851, 570, on Rappaport's award of the Golden Cross of Merit with the Crown (das goldene Verdienstkreuz mit der Krone).

46 I thank Dr. Sergey Kravtsov for bringing this timeline to my attention.

Isaac Epstein and Adam Barach: New leaders of the Jewish hospital

Isaac Epstein (1790–1859) was born in Lviv where his father Mayer was a merchant.[47] Isaac began studying philosophy at Lemberger Lyceum at the age of fourteen (fig. 1.9), making him one of the youngest students there. Two years later, as required of those who wished to progress toward academic degrees, he moved to Vienna to complete his third year of premedical studies at the university there. In 1807, when Isaac Epstein finally registered at the faculty of medicine, he was one of the two Jewish students from Galicia. The only other at the time was Moses Mahl (1781–1823), who would graduate the following year, becoming the first Galician Jew with a doctoral degree from Vienna. The connection between the two men went beyond a casual encounter in Vienna, as Mahl was already married to Isaac Epstein's sister.[48]

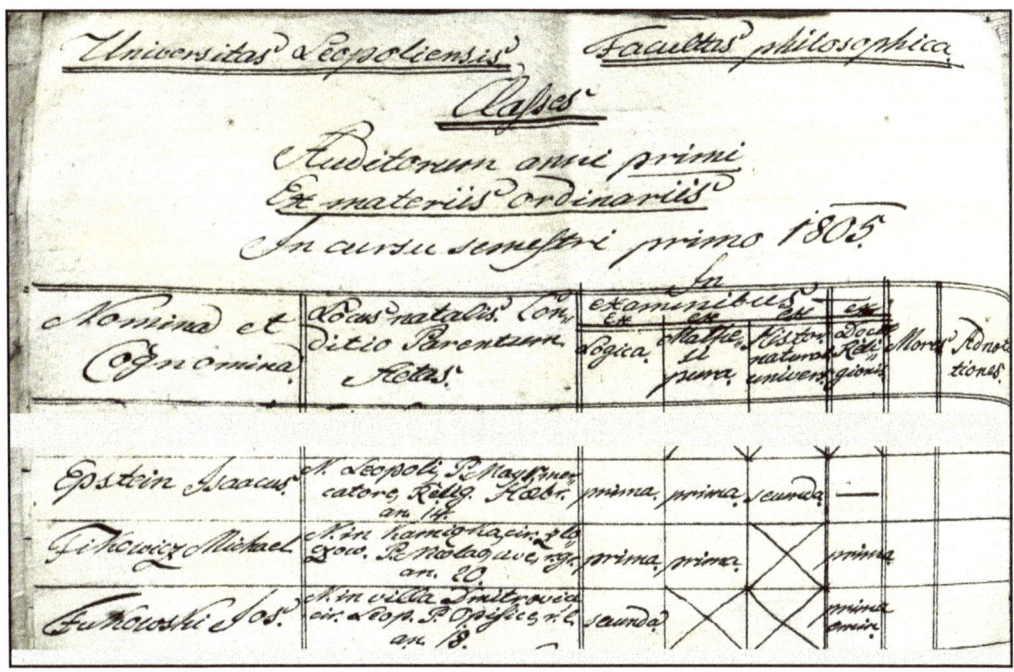

Figure 1.9. Isaac Epstein at Lviv University, 1805. Epstein (the third from the bottom), a first-year student at the Faculty of Philosophy, passed the examinations in logic, mathematics, natural history, and was exempted from studying Christian religious doctrine. A section of the record page. DALO, fond 26, op. 15, spr. 683, f. 578.

---

47 TsDIAL, fond 146, op. 85, spr. 1903, f. 106, Jüdische Normalschulen; Mayer Epstein might have briefly worked as a teacher in a German Jewish school in Lviv.
48 DALO, fond 26, op. 15, spr. 683, f. 461, 497, 503, Lviv University, Classes Auditorum Philosophiae, 1784–1809 (1801–1802, Mahl); fond 26, op. 15, spr. 683, f. 578, 579 (1805, Epstein) and fond 26, op. 15, spr. 685, f. 4, 31, 53, Classes Auditorum Philiosophiae (1805–1806, Epstein); UAW, Med1/14, f. 109, Rigorosenprotokoll, and Med9/5, f. 110, Promotionsprotokoll (1806–1808, Mahl); and TsDIAL, fond 701, op. 2, spr. 29, f. 180, Evidenzbuch, Lea Epstein was the wife of Moses Mahl. He practiced medicine in Lviv (1809–1813), then moved to Brody.

These were precarious times, as Napoleon's armies were marching through Europe. In 1809, Vienna was occupied by the French; the same year, the Austrian army withdrew from a large part of Galicia. Lviv was briefly overrun by Polish insurgents, only to be later occupied by Russian troops. Despite the instability over the next few years, Isaac Epstein persevered. In 1813, when the threat of another French attack had largely abated, he passed his final examinations (*Rigorosen*). The next year, he successfully defended his doctoral dissertation in Vienna and received the doctoral degree in medicine (fig. 1.10). He was one of nine graduates in 1814, five of whom would become university professors in Budapest, Cluj, Innsbruck, and Vienna.[49]

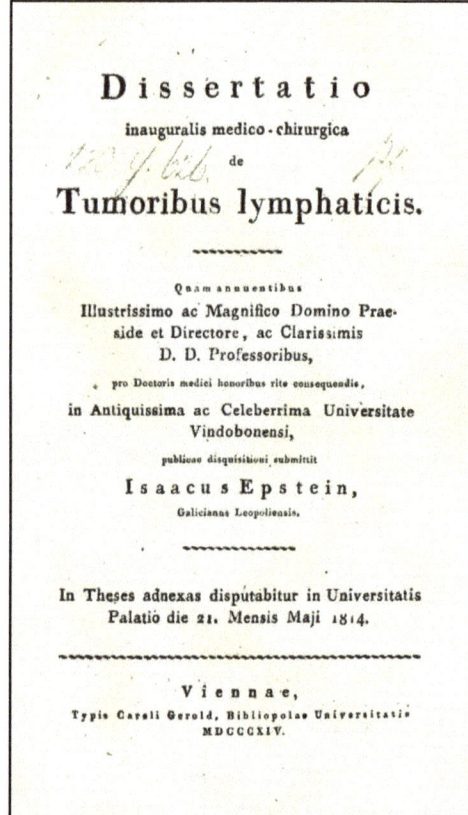 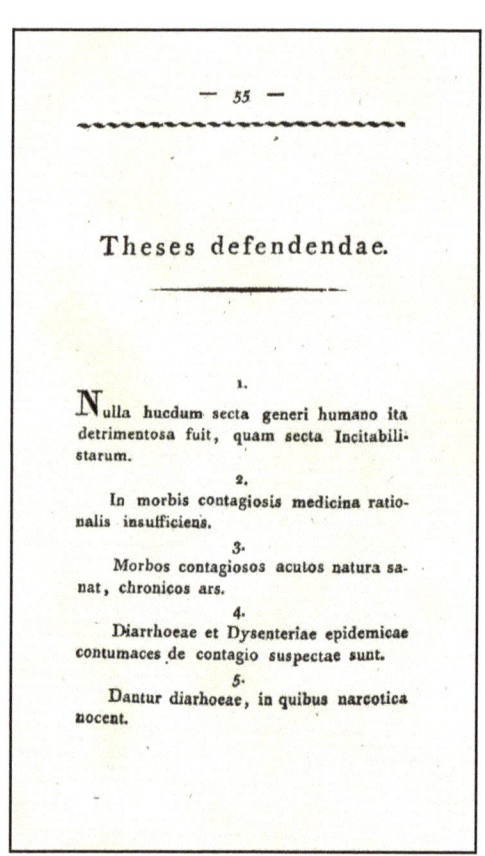

Figure 1.10. Isaac Epstein, *Galicianus Leopoliensis*, at Vienna University, 1814. Left: the cover page of the doctoral dissertation with the date and the place of a public defense of the thesis; the dissertation "Lymphatic Tumors" was written in Latin. Right: the last two pages (with one shown) listed fourteen questions on which the doctoral candidate was questioned. ÖNB, 144333-A.

---

49 Isaacus Epstein, *Dissertatio inauguralis medico-chirurgica de Tumoribus lymphaticis* (Vienna: Bibliopolae Universitatis, 1814), 1–56; *Taschenbuch der Wiener Universität für das Jahr 1815* (Vienna: Gerold, 1815), 121–122, 133–134, for the listing of graduates from 1814.

Shortly after returning home, Dr. Epstein married Dina Waringer in 1815. Dina was the daughter of Isaac Waringer (1741–1817), the administrator and benefactor of the Jewish hospital (see the table on page 37). With so few Jewish doctors present when this institution opened in 1804, the authorities had initially placed it under the oversight of a Polish physician, Ferdinand Stecher von Sebenitz (1779–1857), who was appointed as the Jewish community physician (*Physikus der jüdischen Gemeinde*) and the first medical director of the hospital.[50]

With Epstein's return to Galicia, the situation was about to change. In the eyes of the Habsburg bureaucracy, he was a "model Jew," a professional brought up under the influence of the German language and educated in Vienna. Perhaps not surprisingly, he became the first Jewish physician in chief (*Primararzt*) of the hospital in 1815. For a number of years, he worked as the only full-time physician at the hospital, attending to the needs of about three hundred patients, who were admitted to the ward every year, not to mention making house calls. Under Epstein's watch, the institution would expand, especially during the typhus and cholera epidemics when new facilities were added to care for additional patients.[51]

Primararzt Epstein also pursued nonmedical interests, becoming an early supporter of the plans to erect a new synagogue. He participated in the first planning meeting and signed the founding document (just below the signature of Jacob Rappaport). When the authorities hesitated to issue permission for the synagogue's construction, Epstein coauthored a critical document that provided social and financial justification in support of the initiative.[52]

In 1847, a new leader of the Jewish Hospital emerged. Adam (Ascher) Barach (1803–1867), who succeeded Epstein as physician-in-chief, was part of the same urban circle of Haskalah in Lviv. He also studied at Vienna University, but unlike Epstein, Adam Barach graduated together with three other Jewish students from Galicia in 1831/1832 (fig. 1.11).[53]

Barach was part of the close-knit group of Jewish professionals in Lviv—they socialized together, shared similar interests, and were often connected through marriages. He was married to Nanette (Nina) Rappaport, the daughter of Jacob Rappaport. Barach followed in the footsteps of his accomplished father-in-law, publishing his own observations on the medicinal value of the mineral springs in Galicia—the work that earned him imperial citation in 1843. Later in life, he changed his name to the hyphenated "Barach-Rappaport" as a sign of respect for his father-in-law, the scion of physicians in the city.

---

50 TsDIAL, fond 701, op. 2, spr. 29, f. 155, Evidenzbuch, for the Isaac and Dina Epstein household and their eleven children; Henryk Mehrer, *Szpital lwowskiej gminy wyznaniowej izraelickiej fundacyi Maurycego Lazarusa* (Lwów: Szpital Lwowskiej Gminy Wyzn. Izraelickiej, 1906), 17–20, 24, on Isaac Waringer. Ferdinand Stecher was born in Sambir (Sambor), graduated from Vienna University in 1800 (UAW, Med1/13, f. 652).
51 Mehrer, *Szpital lwowskiej gminy*, 24–28, 36.
52 Bałaban, *Historia lwowskiej synagogi*, xvi, 18–19, 25–26, the petition of August 29, 1842.
53 "Doctoren der Medicin," *Wiener Zeitung*, October 12, 1832, 943, on Lazar Dubs, Salomon Piepes, and Abraham Weinreb. For Adam Barach records, UAW, Med16/20, f. 85, Rigorosenprotokoll and Med11/1, f. 264, Promotionsprotokoll, doctoral degree granted December 12, 1831.

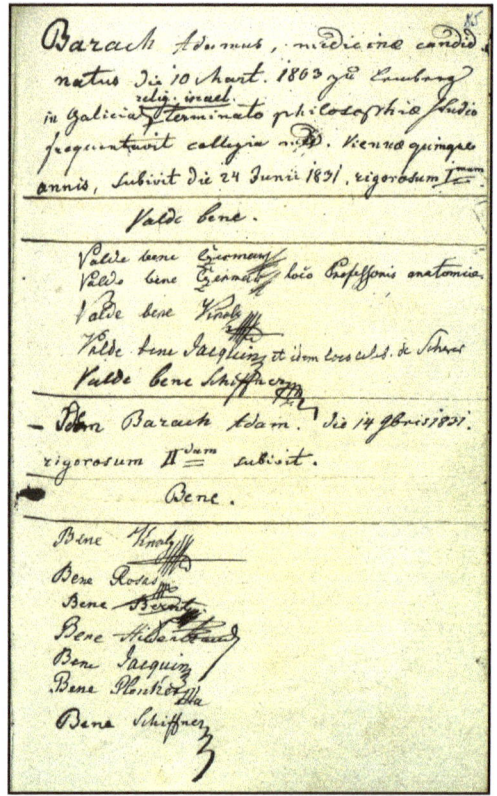 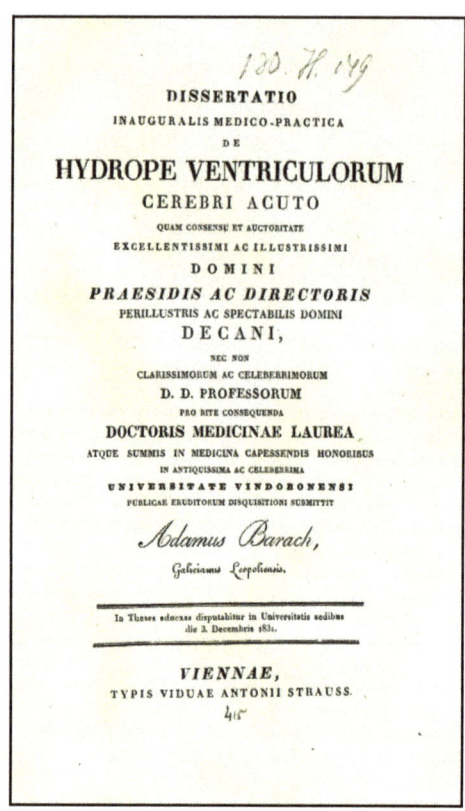

Figure 1.11. Adam Barach, *Galicianus Leopoliensis*, at Vienna University, 1831. Left: the record of two final oral examinations (*Rigorosen*) before the professorial faculty, showing the grades and signatures of the examiners, June and November. UAW, Med16.20, f. 85. Right: the cover page of the doctoral thesis "Acute Hydrocephalus of the Brain," defended in December; it was dedicated to Barach's parents (*parentibus optimis*). ÖNB, 144644-B.

He was also active in philanthropy, served on the Lviv Jewish Community Council, and wrote articles on popular subjects for periodicals in Vienna. After twenty years as director of the Jewish hospital, Adam Barach-Rappaport died of typhus, likely contracted through his professional duties (fig. 1.12).[54]

Moritz Rappaport: Multiculturalist

Moritz (Markus) Rappaport (1808–1880) was born in Lviv.[55] His father was a merchant and early proponent of the Jewish Enlightenment, though his mother remained firmly Orthodox. Moritz was first sent to Vienna, where he attended a prestigious Catholic

---

54 "Wien," *Wiener Zeitung*, March 1, 1843, 453, on the imperial decoration; [no first name] Mahl, "Das neuerrichtete israelitische Waisenhaus in Lemberg," *Lemberger Zeitung*, June 9, 1842, 333–334, on the community work; "Anzeige," *Wiener Zeitung*, September 25, 1847, 416, on the name change; "Tagesneuigkeiten," *Neues Fremden-Blatt*, April 7, 1867, 4, the obituary.
55 No relation to Jacob Rappaport mentioned above.

gymnasium (the Schottengymnasium) and then enrolled in the university. Ultimately, like hundreds of other Galician Jews, Rappaport completed his medical studies at the University of Pest in Hungary (fig. 1.13).[56] After graduating as a doctor of medicine in 1833, he returned to Lviv, where he began working at the Jewish hospital, which was, at that time, still under the direction of Isaac Epstein. Much later in his professional career, Moritz Rappaport succeeded Adam Barach as the next physician in chief, remaining in this position from 1867 to 1872.

Rappaport had begun writing poetry during his time in Vienna—a passion that continued throughout his life. In Lviv, he edited the German-language literary supplement *Leseblätter*. In 1842, his epic poem on biblical themes was his first to earn wider public recognition. Rappaport proved to be a versatile poet. At the outset of the 1848 revolution in the Austrian Empire, he began writing verses in support of political reforms.[57] But he became best known for the epic *Bajazzo*, which in subtle ways, captured the beginning of a cultural shift among his Jewish brethren. It was composed in the context of a failing insurgency in Congress Poland that reflected the Polish quest for independence from Russia in 1863. Rappaport wrote poignantly:

> Passion from the Slavs set my soul ablaze. . . . How nostalgia filled my heart at soft moans of the Sarmathians [Poles], how the spirit rose heavenward at my father's utterances. . . . To be both a Pole and a Jew is a double crown of melancholy![58]

The Jewish poet-physician from Galicia—immersed in Austrian culture and recognized as an acclaimed "German" poet—was identifying himself through his verses with the national aspirations of his neighbors, the ethnic Poles. Rappaport was also credited with German translations of the works of Polish literary classics, making them accessible to many Jews. One of his plays (*Esterka*) captured well the fluidity with which he moved between the different cultural milieus of Galicia—this time, the subject was a fabled love affair between a Polish king and a local Jewish woman. Beginning in 1872, Moritz Rappaport, suffering from a near complete blindness, lived in Vienna where he later died.

---

56 Karl Emil Franzos, "Moritz Rappaport," *Allgemeine Jüdische Zeitung*, October 8, 1892, 485, on studies in the gymnasium and the editorship of Leseblätter (1840–1847); SEL, 50/a, Miscellanea, Historiae Morborum H.M. 570, 50a and vol. 1, f. 192, Album Medicorum, medical degree received June 28, 1833.

57 "Literarisches," *Wiener Zeitschrift*, March 5, 1839, unnumbered pages, announcing Rappaport's epic poem Moses in the "Allgemeines Notizenblatt" section; Heinrich Kurz, *Geschichte der neusten deutschen Literatur mit ausgewählten Stücken aus der Werken der vorzüglichsten Schriftsteller*, vol 4 (Leipzig: B. G. Teubner, 1881), 398–400, on Rappaport's literary works.

58 Adapted from Joseph L. Lichten, "Notes on the Assimilation and Acculturation of Jews in Poland: 1863–1943," in *The Jews in Poland*, ed. Chimen Abramsky, Maciej Jachimczyk, and Antony Polonsky (Oxford: Basil Blackwell, 1986), 109.

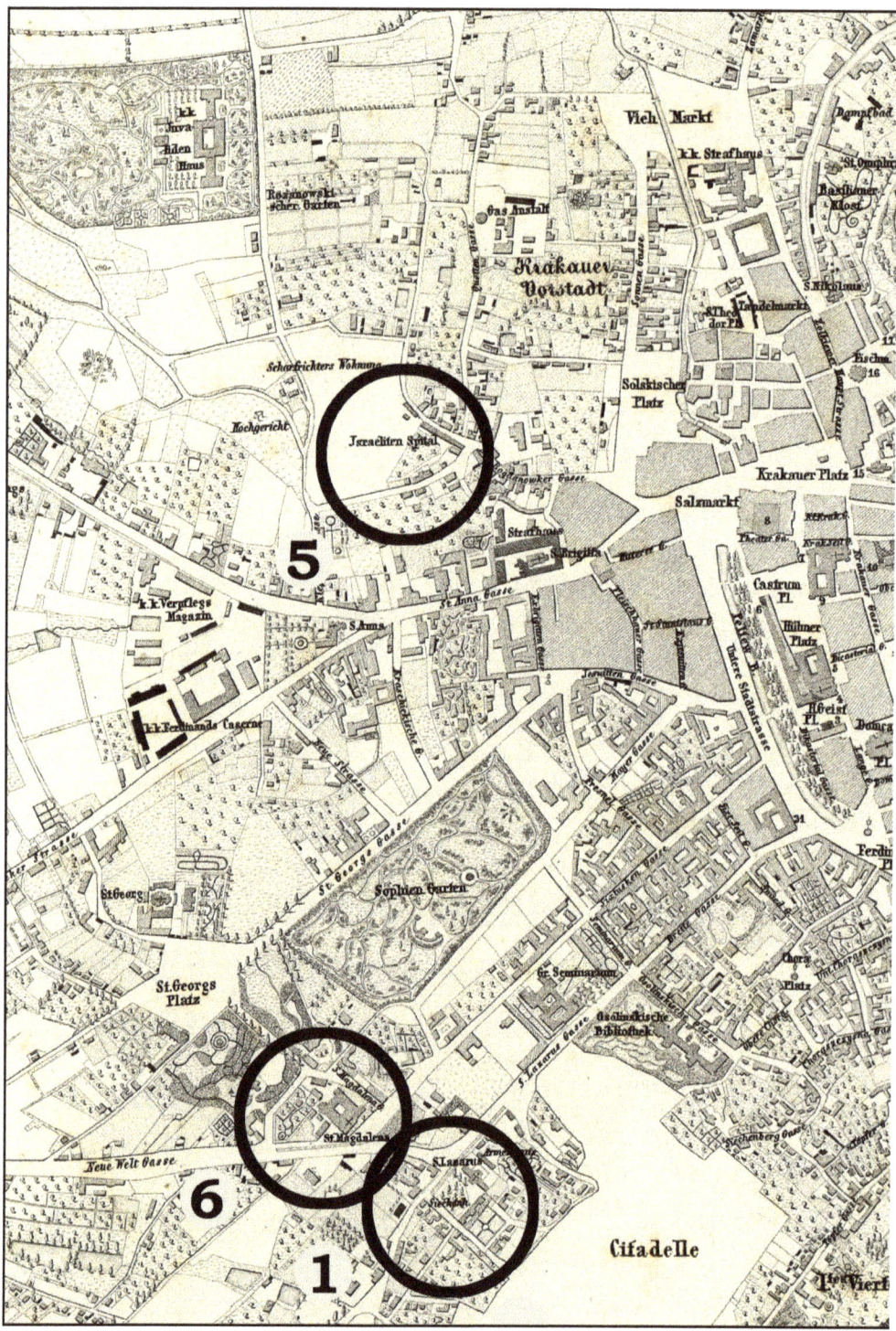

Figure 1.12. Map of Lviv, 1855. The added circles denote Lviv's hospitals in the nineteenth century. (1) St. Lazarus Hospital; (2) Sisters of Mercy Hospital; (3) General Hospital; (4) Military Hospital; (5) Jewish Hospital (Israeliten Spital) in the Kraków suburb (Krakauer Vorstadt); (6) St. Magdalene Hospital; and (7) St. Sophia Hospital (the location after 1880); see table for details. A section of the city map from *Administrativ Karte von den Königreichen Galizien und Lodomerien*. BJ, 122 V, Blatt 24.

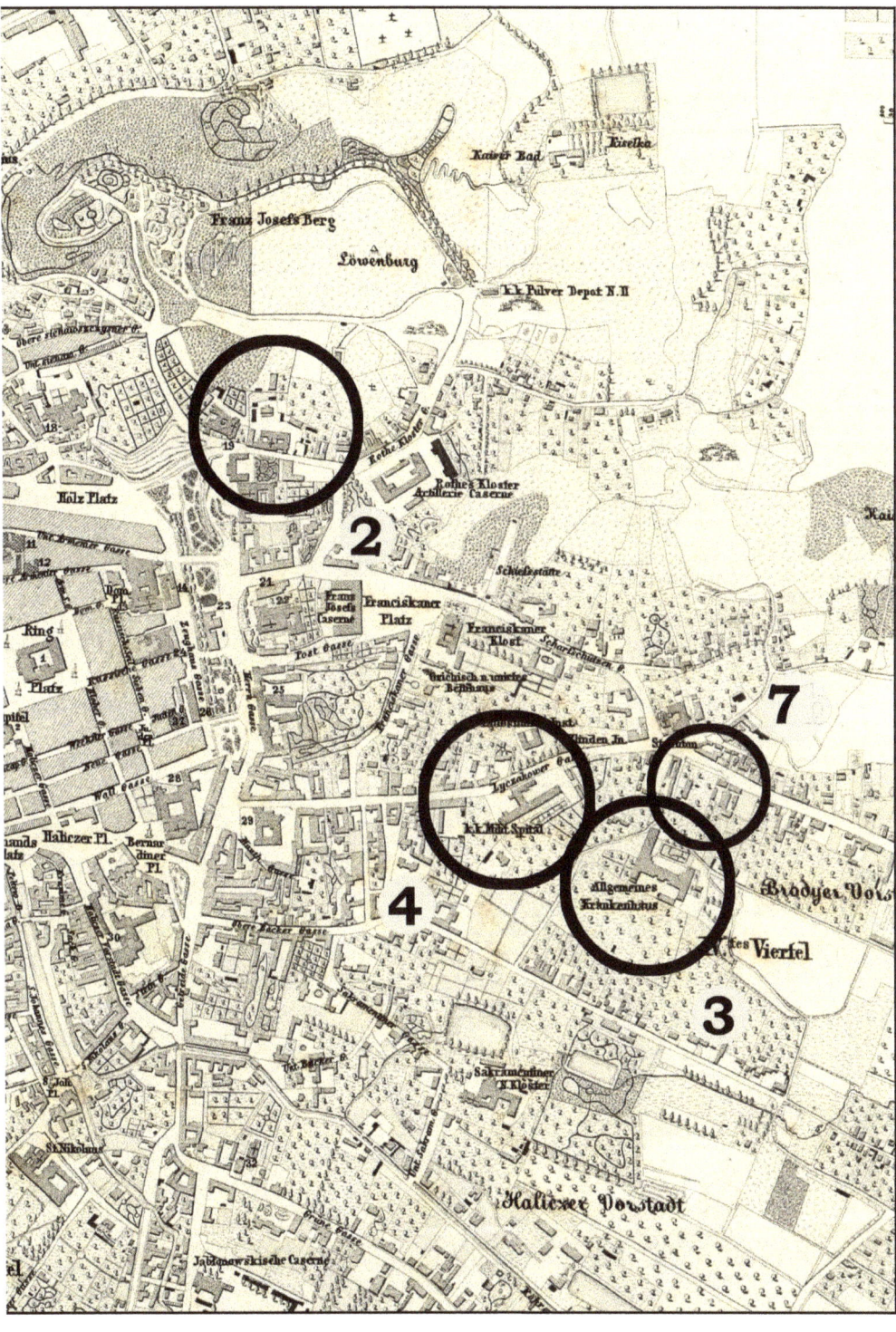

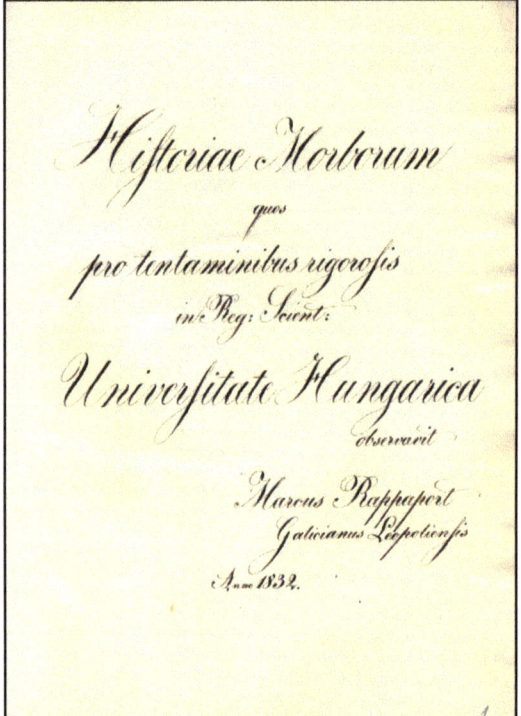 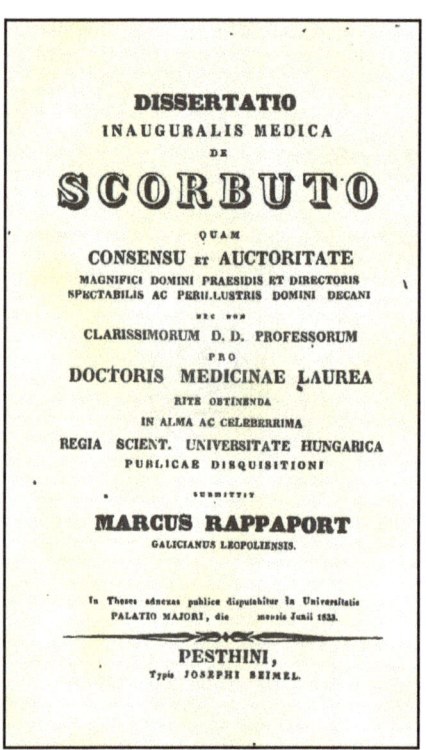

Figure 1.13. Moritz (Marcus) Rappaport, *Galicianus Leopoliensis*, at Pest University, 1832–1833. Left: A *Historiae Morborum*, a detailed report of symptoms, diagnosis and recommended treatments written in Latin was a required submission during the first final examination. SEL H.M. 570, 50/a. Right: the cover page of the doctoral thesis "Scorbuto" (Scurvy), defended by Rappaport in June 1833. OSZK, CV225.22.1833.

Entering the new century

At the end of the nineteenth century, Haskalah's optimistic message that education and German acculturation would make Jews accepted in society lost its appeal. The rise of national movements, the resurgence of antisemitism, and the changes in Galicia, where German-language education yielded to Polish-language schools, caused younger generations to gravitate in new directions. In the multiethnic society, some Jews adopted the dominant Polish cultural identity, a smaller number were attracted to the Ukrainian side, and others were drawn to the Jewish national movement. These trends also affected the new generation of Jewish physicians in Galicia.

In 1894, after a long hiatus, the faculty of medicine was restored at Lviv University. Emperor Franz Joseph attended the ceremony during his visit to the city on the occasion of the national fair. In the first graduating class of 1900, one third of the medical degrees were conferred on new Jewish physicians.[59] Among them were Marek Reichenstein (1876–1932)

---

59 After nonacademic surgery studies were phased out in 1873–1875, the medical faculty was reconstituted as part of the philosophy department in 1894; it became a separate faculty in 1896. For the first graduating class, see DALO, fond 26, op. 15, spr. 963, Lviv University; nine out of twenty-seven graduates were Jewish.

and Natan Schneider (1873–1941), who would remain close, marrying sisters whose lives reflected the changing times as well. Marek Reichenstein married Adelle Kalmus in 1903, while two years later his former classmate Nathan Schneider married Maria Kalmus.[60]

Marek Reichenstein initially worked at the university clinic and later became a hematologist in Lviv. After World War I, he increasingly devoted himself to collecting and researching art. Among his eclectic repository of artifacts were Polish woodcuts and foreign graphics, rare books, and an array of Judaica, including illuminated Italian Jewish marriage contracts (*ketubbot*). Whether supporting art and book exhibits with items from his collection or engaging in efforts to document the Jewish artistic heritage of Galicia, Reichenstein was part of many cultural initiatives. His wife Adelle (Ada), who was active in Zionist women's organizations, continued her husband's mission after his death.[61] When the long-awaited Jewish Museum opened in Lviv in 1934, most of the Judaica from the Reichenstein collection was put on a permanent display there.[62]

Trailblazing women

Throughout the centuries, "wise women" were sought for health-related advice; many women were caregivers for the sick and assisted during labor.[63] In the early period of Austrian Galicia, women took midwifery courses in Lviv and in other towns (fig. 1.14). Jewish female students from Galicia could be also found in Hungary, where they earned required credentials. Among those were Cecilia Braun from Brody and Emilia Perl from Łańcut who attended Pest University in 1835 and 1838, respectively.[64] These midwives were sometimes the wives of local surgeons, and they and their husbands provided the only available medical services in smaller communities in Galicia.

Until the end of the nineteenth century, however, women could not advance further in medical careers. They were legally precluded from earning university degrees in Austria-Hungary. When Rosa Welt (1857–1938) from Bukovina (a province in the Austro-Hungarian Empire), completed her medical studies in Switzerland in 1878, she became the first woman physician in her home country. Even though several newspapers reported on her accomplishment, she was unable to practice medicine in Austria-Hungary because of her gender. As a result, Rosa Welt emigrated to the United States.[65]

---

60 I thank Raymund Minkus for the information on both sisters.
61 Adelle Reichenstein co-founded the Union of Jewish Women in 1925 and the Women's International Zionist Organization in 1929.
62 Sergey R. Kravtsov, "Marek Reichenstein: Collector and His Collection," in *Jewish Marriage Contracts: Collection of Ketubbot in the Borys Voznytsky National Art Gallery of Lviv*, ed. Vita Susak (Lviv: Borys Voznytsky National Art Gallery of Lviv and Center for Urban History of East Central Europe, 2015), 11–27, for an excellent biography of Reichenstein and a description of his collection.
63 Nimrod Zinger, "Tuviya Cohen and the Medical Marketplace in the Early Modern Period," *Korot* 20 (2009–2010): 72–77, on the societal, rabbinic, and medical establishment's attitudes toward "wise women."
64 Kempel-Kürsinger, *Handbuch der Gesetzkunde*, 4:528–531, on regulations regarding midwives; SEL, 1/d, vols. 28, 34, Libri classificationum, records of Jewish midwifery students.
65 In 1919, Rosa Welt moved from the United States to Palestine where she became a champion of women's rights.

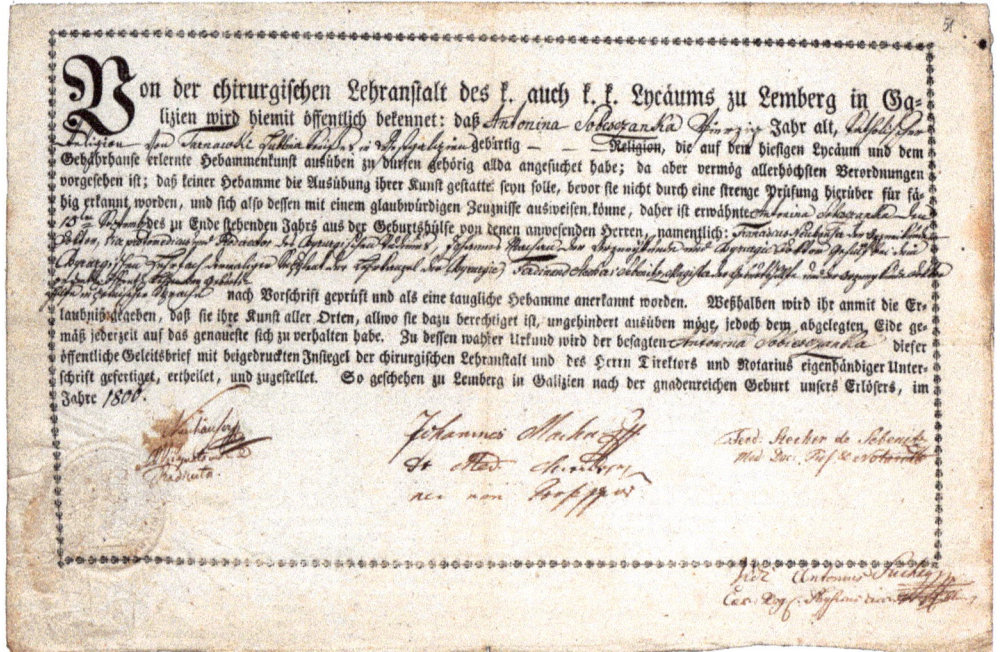

Figure 1.14. Diploma certificate of a midwife issued by the surgical school (*chirurgischen Lehranstalt*) in Lviv, 1806. It was co-signed by Ferdinand Stecher von Sebenitz (right), the director of the Jewish Hospital, 1804–1815. APL, 35/22/0/4.6.1.4/2247, f. 51.

Beginning in 1896, women doctors educated abroad, mainly in Switzerland, could obtain permission to practice medicine in Austria. The following year, the first female students were also admitted to study philosophy, with the right to earn doctoral degrees at the universities in Austria-Hungary.[66] At the same time, "academic courses for women" taught by university professors became available in Galicia. In January 1897, more than 350 women enrolled in a series of lectures in Lviv alone. Similar initiatives sprung up in other cities. Even though the participants received no formal educational credits or employment benefits, the women's response sent a clear message about their hunger for higher education.[67]

The breakthrough came in 1900 when women were finally permitted to earn medical degrees in Austrian universities.[68] That same year, Maria Kalmus (1879–?), who had been denied admission only a year before, quickly transferred from Zurich to Lviv University. In

---

66 "Betreffend die Nostrification der von Frauen im Auslande erworbenen medicinischen Doctordiploma," *Reichsgesetzblatt*, no. 45 (March 19, 1896): 211–212; "Betreffend die Zulassung von Frauen als ordentliche oder ausser ordentliche Hörerinnen an den philosophischen Facultäten," *Reichsgesetzblatt*, no. 84 (March 23, 1897): 427–428. In special circumstances, women could attend individual lectures in medicine with permission from the professorial faculty.
67 "Towarzystwo kursów akademickich," *Gazeta Lwowska*, April 13, 1897, 4, on the lectures for women.
68 "Betreffend die Zulassung von Frauen zu den medicinischen Studien und zum Doctorate der gesammten Heilkunde," *Reichsgesetzblatt*, no. 149 (September 3, 1900): 379–380, the pharmacy admitted women in 1903. The faculty of law relaxed admissions policies only in 1919.

1904, she became the first woman to graduate as a doctor of general medicine (fig. 1.15).⁶⁹ The event was clearly newsworthy, though the leading dailies in Lviv mistook Maria for her sister, Adelle Kalmus, who had earned the first doctorate from the faculty of philosophy a year before. Maria Schneider (née Kalmus) became an obstetrician-gynecologist, who was also involved in social work on behalf of patients. For years, she remained a steadfast champion of Jewish medical students at the university. She retired from clinical practice in 1936.⁷⁰

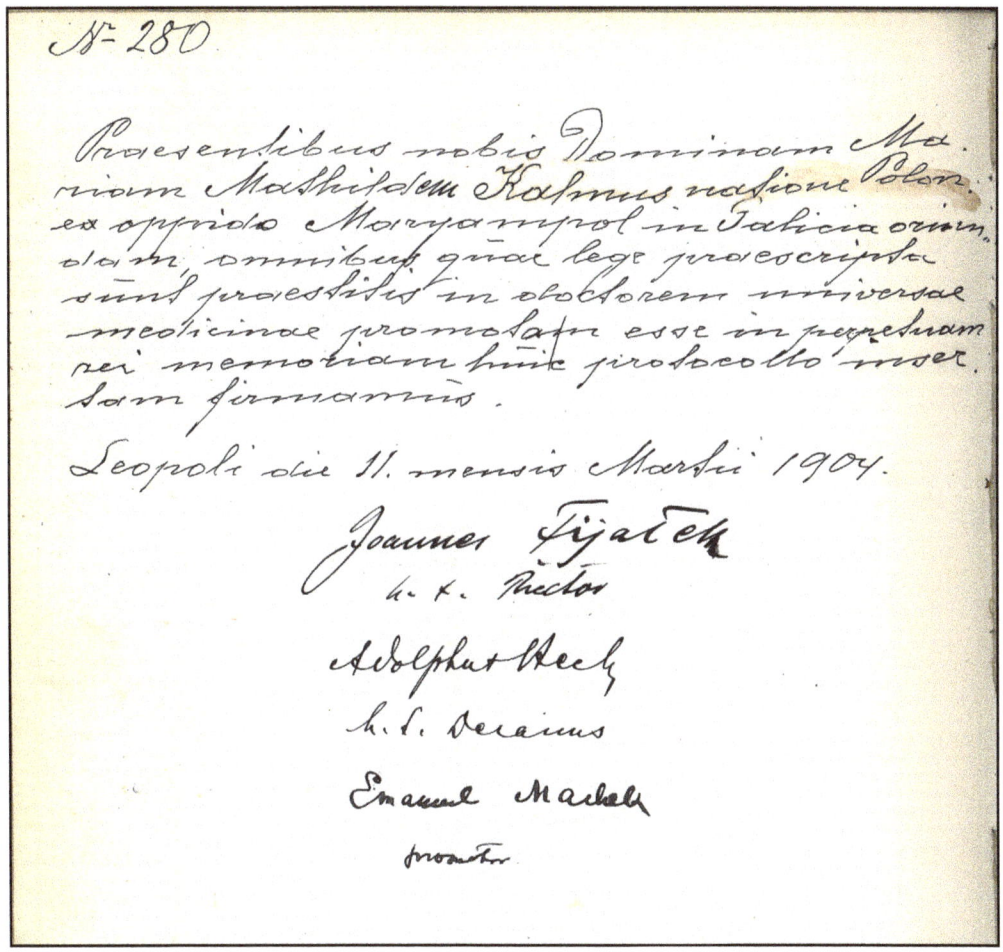

Figure 1.15. Maria Mathilda Kalmus promoted to the doctor of general medicine. She became the first female physician who graduated at Lviv University, March 11, 1904. DALO, fond 26, op. 15, spr. 1345.

---

69 DALO, fond 26, op. 15, spr. 1345, f. not numbered, Lviv University, Album Promotionum, 1900–1904; Jadwiga Suchmiel, Żydówki ze stopniem doktora wszech nauk lekarskich oraz doktora filozofii na Universytecie Jagiellońskim do czasów II Rzeczypospolitej (Częstochowa: WSP, 1997), 25–26, 31–33; at Jagiellonian University, Helena Donhajser-Sikorska (non-Jewish) was the first to complete medical studies in 1906. The Jewish women, Maria Horowitz, Regina Korngold, and Waleria Lustgarten, graduated in 1907.

70 "Kronika," Kurjer lwowski, March 11, 1904, 4; "O dziecko żydowskie," Chwila, April 26, 1922, 5, on social initiatives; "Sprawozdanie," Trybuna Akademicka, January 1933, 16; and "Kronika," Chwila, March 9, 1934, 12, on support of Jewish students; Marek Redner, "Recollections on the Life and Martyrdom of Jewish Medical Doctors in the Lvov Ghetto," unpublished, 46; her husband, Natan Schneider, was killed in July 1941 in Lviv.

For some women, a career in medicine meant the continuation of a long family tradition that until recently was only available to men. In 1905, Matylda Lateiner (1880–1961) became the second woman to graduate with a medical degree in Lviv (fig. 1.16).[71] Her grandfather and father were physicians in Galicia, as were other members from the extended Lateiner family. Matylda, a rising star in her own right, was the first woman physician to join the academic faculty in Lviv. Before World War I, she moved to Vienna. In the interwar period, she and her husband, Dr. Ernst Mayerhofer, settled in Zagreb (then in Yugoslavia), where they survived the war.

The story of Franciszka Fuchs (1881–1942) is very different. In some ways, her experience resembled the lives of Isaac Epstein, Adam Barach-Rappaport, and Moritz Rappaport. Like those men, she was from Lviv and was also among the "first" when she became a Jewish woman physician in 1906.[72] Fanny, as she was known in her youth, worked at the outpatient clinic of the new Jewish hospital in Lviv—the Maurycy Lazarus Foundation Israelite Hospital—on Rappaport Street. She was considered "one of the most popular personalities" among women doctors in the prewar city. During the Holocaust, as one of her colleagues later recalled, she worked tirelessly as a physician in the ghetto, exuding empathy to others even under the most harrowing circumstances. Franciszka Reich (née Fuchs) was murdered in August 1942.[73]

***

There were many facets to the experience of Jewish medical practitioners. Before the First Partition of Poland, some Jews from Galicia gained university education studying medicine in culturally transforming settings, first in Italy and later in Germany. At the end of the eighteenth century, the reforms introduced by Emperor Joseph II opened the Habsburg schools to Jews. This slowly increased the number of Jewish physicians in Austrian Galicia, who by virtue of their profession, moved with greater ease across the societal divisions existing at the time.

Early nineteenth-century Jewish physicians shared a common cultural orientation, with a new sense of aesthetics, and kinship with other members of the Galician Haskalah. They all supported secular education and were often proponents of religious reforms, joining the Progressive movement. A number of physicians served on Jewish Community Councils and represented their coreligionists with the authorities. Some of them became recognized for their literary talents—their choice of German, Hebrew, or Polish reflected both the multiethnic society and the shifting political changes in Galicia. After political and legal emancipation was granted to all citizens of the Austrian part (Cisleithania) of the Austro-Hungarian Empire in 1867, Jewish participation in university education greatly

---

71 DALO, fond 26, op. 15, spr. 963, f. 20, Lviv University, Protokół egzaminów ścisłych, 1897–1922; the university records indicate Lateiner's excellent academic performance during her medical studies.
72 DALO, fond 26, op. 15, spr. 1346, f. 164, Lviv University, Album Promotionum, 1904–1907.
73 "Z kroniki żałobnej," *Chwila*, April 6, 1927, 6; Franciszka Fuchs was married to Alfred Reich, a German language professor and Zionist who died in 1927; Redner, "Recollections on the Life and Martyrdom," 44, for recollections about Franciszka Fuchs-Reich.

accelerated. Throughout this period, doctors affiliated with the Jewish hospital in Lviv were harbingers of cultural trends and new secular identities making inroads into the Jewish community at large.

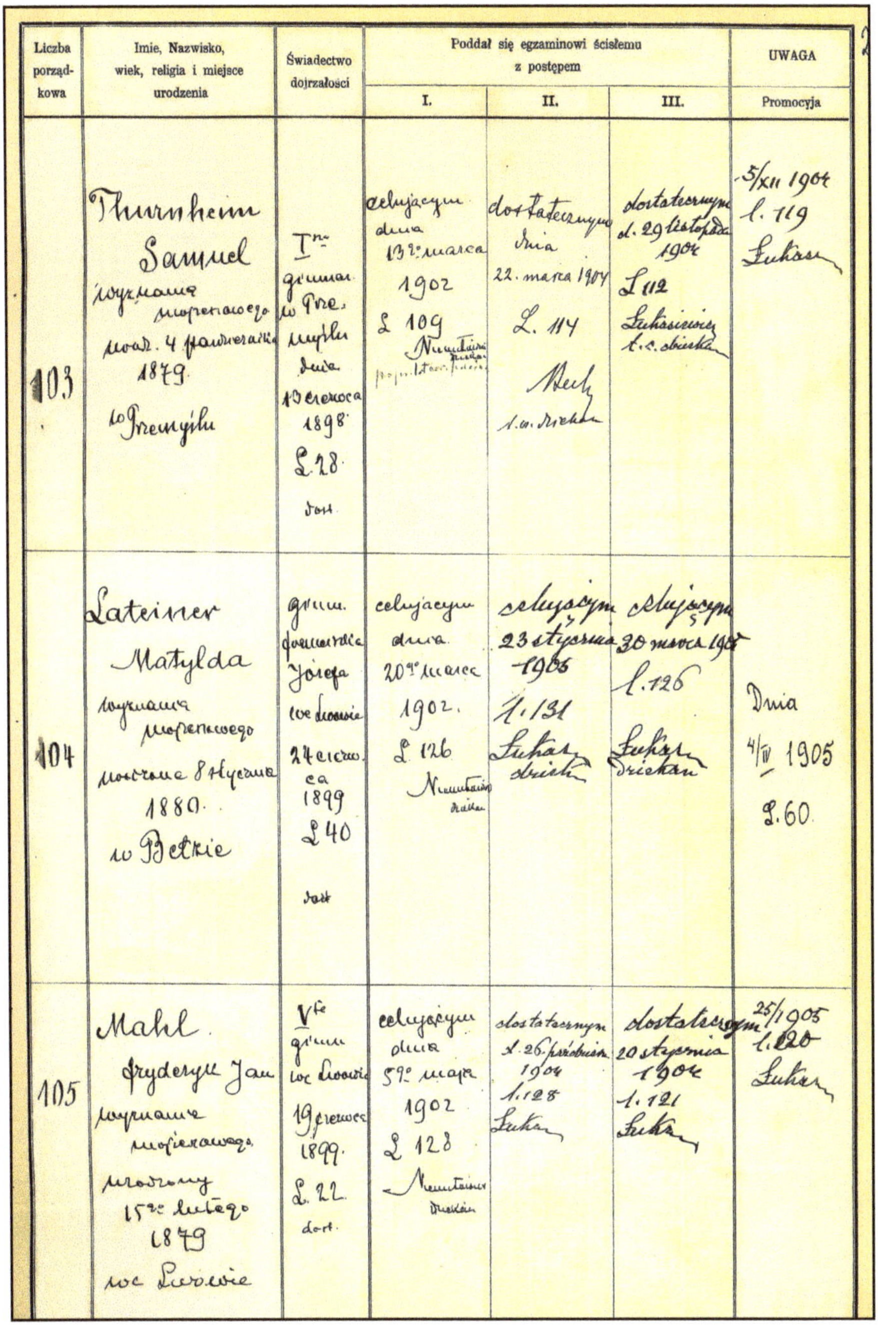

Figure 1.16. Samuel Thurnheim (top), Matylda Lateiner (middle), and Fryderyk Jan Mahl (bottom), three Jewish medical students at Lviv University. Matylda Lateiner passed with distinction three final examinations and became the second female physician who graduated from the university, April 4, 1905. DALO, fond 26, op. 15, spr. 963, f. 20.

At the beginning of the twentieth century, the arrival of Jewish women physicians occurred in a different context. The opening of the universities to women in the Austro-Hungarian Empire was no longer part of the state's effort to integrate the Jewish minority in the broader society. Instead, it was an initial step toward "gender emancipation." For many women, and Jewish women in particular, access to higher education gave them the opportunity to modernize their lives. By the end of Austrian Galicia in 1918, about 30% of all students were Jewish in the two universities there. Jewish women students accounted for approximately half of all the women studying medicine.[74] These numbers reflected their rapid embrace of a new social paradigm.

---

74 Suchmiel, Żydówki, 10, 12, the large number of women led to a 15% cap on their admissions in 1918.

TABLE. Hospitals in nineteenth-century Lviv

Hospital	Established	Historical Location	Comments
St. Lazarus Hospital	1618	Halicz district (I) 1 Św. Łazarz St.	Served indigent patients 1787: became municipal hospital to replace defunct hospitals in the city
Sisters of Mercy Hospital	1741	Żółkiew district (III) 1 Teatyńska St.	Served indigent patients and provided hospice care 1783: the orphanage moved to a building of the former Reformed Franciscans Order
General Hospital	1783	Łyczaków district (IV) 7 Głowiński St.	Founded by Joseph II in the former Collegium Nobilium of the Piarists 1805–1873: teaching hospital for surgeons and midwives 1829: Jews not admitted to the General Hospital 1874: all patients admitted regardless of social status, ethnicity, or religion
Military Hospital	1784	Łyczaków district (IV) 26 Łyczakowska St.	The building complex of the former Bonifrater Order
Jewish Hospital	1804	Kraków district (II) 2 Rappaport St.	Founded with support of Isaac Waringer 1831: cholera and typhus treatment facilities added 1838: subsidized by estate taxes, cemetery fees, and endowments 1903: the Maurycy Lazarus Foundation Israelite Hospital opened
St. Magdalene Hospital	1831	Kraków district (II) 4 Nowy Świat St.	Cholera hospital in the former Dominican cloister 1841–1923: a women's correctional institution
St. Sophia Hospital	1845	Kraków district (II) 24 Nowy Świat St.	Children hospital founded by the women's association
		Łyczaków district (IV) 42 Łyczakowska St.	1880: in a new location 1910: part of the General Hospital

Sources: city districts (with Roman numerals) according to maps 1855, 1895; the former Brody district is named here the Łyczaków district. The streets: *Skorowidz nowych i dawnych numerów realności* (Lwów: Karol Wild, 1872), with modifications for later additions. Other details: Michael Stöger, *Darstellung der gezetzlichen Verfassung der galizischen Judenschaft*, vol. 2 (Lemberg: n.p., 1833), 61n12; Ignacy Chodyniecki, *Historya miasta Lwowa* (Lwów: n.p., 1829), 377, 381, 390, 393, 395–396; Emil Moniak, *Historja kościoła pod wezwaniem św. Marji Magdaleny* (Lwów: n.p., 1927), 13–14; Alfons Schletz, "Historia Sióstr Miłosierdzia," *Nasza Przeszłość* 12 (1960): 63–71; Piotr Franaszek, "Krajowy szpital powszechny we Lwowie," *Zeszyty Naukowe Uniwersytetu Jagiellońskiego* 127 (2000): 122.

Archival Sources

AUJ
S I/505, f. 31.
WL I/84, f. 37.
WL I/86, f. not numbered.
WL I/91, f. not numbered.

DALO
Fond 26, op. 4, spr. 211, f. 147.
Fond 26, op. 15, spr. 683, f. 372, 461, 497, 503, 578–579.
Fond 26, op. 15, spr. 685, f. 4, 31, 53.
Fond 26, op. 15, spr. 963, f. 6, 7, 20, 24.
Fond 26, op. 15, spr. 1345, f. not numbered.
Fond 26, op. 15, spr. 1346, f. 164.
Fond 26, op. 22, spr. 2348, f. 1–3, 8–10.

SEL
H.M. 570, 50/a.
1/f, vol. 1.
1/d, vol. 28.
1/d, vol. 34.

TsDIAL
Fond 146, op. 85, spr. 1903, f. 106.
Fond 701, op. 2, spr. 29, f. 155, 180.

UAW
Med1/13, f. 652.
Med1/14, f. 109.
Med9/5, f. 110.
Med11/1, f. 264.
Med16.20, f. 85.

Bibliography

"Anzeige." *Wiener Zeitung*, September 25, 1847.
Bałaban, Majer. *Historja Żydów w Krakowie i na Kazimierzu 1304–1868*. 2 vols. Kraków: Nadzieja, 1931–1936.
———. *Z historji Żydów w Polsce*. Warszawa: Lewin-Epstein, 1920.

———. "Lekarze żydowscy w dawnej Rzeczypospolitej." In *Żydzi w Polsce odrodzonej*, vol. 1, edited by I. Schiper, A. Tartakower, and A. Hafftka, 289–307. Warszawa: Żydzi w Polsce Odrodzonej, 1932.

———. *Historia lwowskiej synagogi postępowej*. Lwów: Zarząd Synagogi Postępowej, 1937.

Barzilay, Isaac. *Yoseph Shlomo Delmedigo (Yashar of Candia): His Life, Work and Times*. Leiden: E. J. Brill, 1974.

"Betreffend die Nostrification der von Frauen im Auslande erworbenen medicinischen Doctordiploma." *Reichsgesetzblatt für die im Reichsrathe vertretenen Königreiche und Länder*, no. 45 (March 19, 1896): 211–212.

"Betreffend die Praxis der Wundärzte." *Reichsgesetzblatt für die im Reichsrathe vertretenen Königreiche und Länder*, no. 25 (February 17, 1873): 125.

"Betreffend die Zulassung von Frauen als ordentliche oder ausserordentliche Hörerinnen an den philosophischen Facultäten der k.k. Universitäten." *Reichsgesetzblatt für die im Reichsrathe vertretenen Königreiche und Länder*, no. 84 (March 23, 1897): 427–428.

"Betreffend die Zulassung von Frauen zu den medicinischen Studien und zum Doctorate der gesammten Heilkunde." *Reichsgesetzblatt für die im Reichsrathe vertretenen Königreiche und Länder*, no. 149 (September 3, 1900): 379–381.

Bicker, K. B, "Die Verbreitung der Cholera morbus im Jahre 1831." *Hesperus* 1, no. 6–7 (1832): 23–28.

Bylebyl, Jerome J. "The Medical Meaning of Physica." *Osiris* 6, no. 1 (1990): 16–41.

Del Negro, Piero, ed. *The University of Padua: Eight Centuries of History*. Padua: Signumpadova, 2003.

"Die Einführung der neuen Juden-Ordnung betreffend. Allgemeine Ordnung für die gesammte Judenschaft der Königreiche Gallizien und Lodomerien." In *Continuatio Edictorum et Mandatorum Universalium in Regnis Galiciae et Lodomeriae*, 76–121. Lwów: A. Piller, 1776.

"Doctoren der Medicin." *Wiener Zeitung*, October 12, 1832.

Efron, John M. *Medicine and The German Jews: A History*. New Haven: Yale University Press, 2001.

Epstein, Isaacus. *Dissertatio inaugaralis medico-chirurgica de Tumoribus lymphaticis*. Vienna: Bibliopolae Universitatis, 1814.

Franzos, Karl Emil. "Moritz Rappaport." *Allgemeine Jüdische Zeitung*, October 8, 1892.

Friedenwald, Harry. *The Jews and Medicine*. 2 vols. Baltimore: Johns Hopkins Press, 1944.

Garcia-Ballester, Luis, Lolla Ferre, and Eduard Feliu. "Jewish Appreciation of Fourteenth-Century Scholastic Medicine." *Osiris* 6, no. 1, (1990): 85–117.

Gath, Isak N. "The Elusive Karaite Doctor Joseph Ezra Dubitski, the 'Sobieski Hours', and the Myth of Polish Lithuanian Karaite Physicians." *Karaite Archives* 3, no. 1 (2015): 5–35.

Gräffer, Franz. "Rappaport, Jacob." In *Jüdischer Plutarch*, vol. 1, 174–178. Vienna: Ulrich Klopf, 1848.

"Gratis erigitur studium artis Medicae, Chyrurgicae & Obstetricae." In *Continuatio Edictorum et Mandatorum Universalium in Regnis Galiciae et Lodomeriae*, 9–10. Lwów: A. Piller, 1774.

Maria Horodyska. "Wydział Filozoficzny w Uniwersytecie Józefińskim, 1784–1804." PhD diss., Lviv University, 1933.

Kalik, Judith. "Office Holders of the Council of Four Lands, 1595–1764." In *Jewish Self-Government in Eastern Europe*, edited by François Guesnet and Antony Polonsky, Polin: Studies in Polish Jewry, 131–161. London: Littman Library, 2022.

Kempel-Kürsinger, Johann. *Handbuch der Gesetzkunde im Sanitäts- und Medicinal-Gebiethe.* 4 vols. Vienna: k. k. Hof- und Staats-Aerarial Druckerei, 1830–1832.

Kisch, Guido. *Die Prager Universität und die Juden 1348–1848*. Amsterdam: Verlag B. R. Grüner, 1969.

Koren, Nathan. *Jewish Physicians: A Biographical Index*. Jerusalem: Israel Universities Press, 1973.

Korns, Horace Marshall. "Notes on the Medical History of Vienna." *Annals of Medical History* 9, no. 4 (1937): 345–481.

Kratter, Franz. *Briefe über den itzigen Zustand von Galizien*. Vol. 2. Leipzig: G. Ph. Wucherers, 1786.

Kravtsov, Sergey R. "The Progressive Synagogue in Lemberg/Lwów/Lviv: Architecture and Community." In *Jews and Slavs*, vol. 23, edited by Wolf Moskovich, Roman Mnich, and Renata Tarasiuk, 185–214. Jerusalem-Siedlce: The Hebrew University of Jerusalem and Siedlce University of Natural Sciences and Humanities, 2013.

Kravtsov, Sergey R. "Marek Reichenstein: Collector and His Collection." In *Jewish Marriage Contracts: Collection of Ketubbot in the Borys Voznytsky National Art Gallery of Lviv*, edited by Vita Susak, 11–27. Lviv: Borys Voznytsky National Art Gallery of Lviv and Center for Urban History of East Central Europe, 2015.

"Kronika." *Chwila*, March 9, 1934.

"Kronika." *Kurjer lwowski*, March 11, 1904.

Kurz, Heinrich. *Geschichte der neusten deutschen Literatur mit ausgewählten Stücken aus der Werken der vorzüglichsten Schriftsteller*. Vol. 4. Leipzig: Teubner, 1881.

Lichten, Joseph L. "Notes on the Assimilation and Acculturation of Jews in Poland: 1863–1943." In *The Jews in Poland*, edited by Chimen Abramsky, Maciej Jachimczyk, and Antony Polonsky, 106–129. New York: B. Blackwell, 1986.

"Literarisches." *Wiener Zeitschrift*, March 5, 1839.

Mahl [no first name]. "Das neuerrichtete israelitische Waisenhaus in Lemberg." *Lemberger Zeitung*, June 9, 1842.

Mehrer, Henryk. *Szpital lwowskiej gminy wyznaniowej izraelickiej fundacyi Maurycego Lazarusa*. Lwów: Szpital Lwowskiej Gminy Wyzn. Izraelickiej, 1906.

Neuburger, Max. "Die ersten an der Wiener medizinischen Fakultät promovierten Arzte jüdischen Stammes." *Monatschrift für Geschichte und Wissenschaft des Judentums* 26, no. 3 (1918): 219–222.

"O dziecko żydowskie." *Chwila*, April 26, 1922.

"Oesterreichischer Kaiserstaat." *Allgemeine Zeitung des Judenthums*, November 24, 1851.

Petrovsky-Shtern, Yohanan. "The Master of an Evil Name: Hillel Ba'al Shem and his Sefer ha-heshek." *AJS Review* 28, no. 2 (2004): 217–248.

Rappaport, Jacob. "Ueber die Contagiosität der Cholera im Vergleiche zur Pest." *Archiv für medizinische Erfahrung im Gebiete der praktischen Medizin, Chirurgie, Gebrutshülfe und Staatsarzneikunde* 25 (September–October 1831): 867–877.

Redner, Marek. "Recollections on the Life and Martyrdom of Jewish Medical Doctors in the Lvov Ghetto." Unpublished manuscript.

Reichman, Edward. "Notes on the Jewish Renaissance Physician Gabriel Felix: His Grammar Tree and His Family Tree." *Korot* 2 (2019–2020): 339–353.

Richarz, Monika. *German Jews and the University, 1678–1848*. Rochester: Camden House, 2022.

Rosman, M. J. *The Lord's Jews: Magnate-Jewish Relations in the Polish-Lithuanian Commonwealth during the 18th Century*. Cambridge, MA: Harvard University Press, 1990.

Roth, Cecil. "The Qualification of Jewish Physicians in the Middle Ages." *Speculum* 28, no. 4 (1953): 834–843.

Ruderman, David B. *Jewish Thought and Scientific Discovery in Early Modern Europe*. New Haven: Yale University Press, 1995.

"Schreiben eines freundes an seinen freund von Brody in Pohlen." *Wienerisches Diarum*, January 29, 1774.

Shatzky, Jacob. "On Jewish Medical Students of Padua." *Journal of the History of Medicine and Allied Sciences* 5 (Autumn 1950): 444–447.

Śleszkowski, Sebastyan. *Iasne dowody o doktorach żydowskich*. Kraków: 1649.

"Sprawozdanie o działalności tow. medyków żyd. U. J. K. we Lwowie za rok aka. 1931/32." *Trybuna Akademicka*, January 1933.

"Statuit Provinciales Medicos, ex eorumque consilio, praescribit, quid reliqui in usu artis medicae observare debeant." In *Edicta et Mandata Universalia Regnis Galiciae et Lodomeriae*, 45–50. Lwów: J. Piller, 1773.

Suchmiel, Jadwiga. *Żydówki ze stopniem doktora wszech nauk lekarskich oraz doktora filozofii na Uniwersytecie Jagiellońskim do czasów II Rzeczypospolitej*. Częstochowa: WSP, 1997.

Szumowski, Władysław. *Galicia pod względem medycznym za Jędrzeja Krupińskiego pierwszego protomedyka 1772–1783*. Lwów: Towarzystwo Popierania Nauki Polskiej, 1907.

"Tagesneuigkeiten." *Neues Fremden-Blatt*, April 7, 1867.

Taschenbuch der Wiener Universität für das Jahr 1815. Vienna: Gerold, 1815.

"Towarzystwo kursów akademickich dla kobiet." *Gazeta Lwowska*, April 13, 1897.

Warchał, Jan. "Żydzi polscy na uniwersytecie padewskim." *Kwartalnik poświęcony badaniu przeszłości Żydów w Polsce* 1, no. 3 (1913): 37–72.

"Wien." *Wiener Zeitung*, March 1, 1843.

Wischnitzer, Mark. *A History of Jewish Crafts and Guilds*. New York: Davide Publishers, 1965.

Wolf, Gerson. *Studies zur Jubelfeier der Wiener Univesität im Jahre 1865*. Vienna: Herzfeld & Bauer, 1865.

"Z kroniki żałobnej." *Chwila*, April 6, 1927.

Zalewski, Andrew. "Becoming Habsburg Galitzianers." *Galitzianer* 26, no. 3 (2019): 12–17.

———. "The First Habsburg Census." *Galitzianer* 26, no. 4 (2019): 6–10

———. *Galician Portraits: In Search of Jewish Roots*. Jenkintown: Thelzo Press, 2014.

Zinger, Nimrod. "Tuviya Cohen and the Medical Marketplace in the Early Modern Period." *Korot* 20 (2009–2010): 67–95.

Chapter 2

Maurycy Lazarus, Founder of the Jewish Hospital, and His Family[*]

Ewa Herbst

At the end of the nineteenth century the Jewish community of Lviv desperately needed a new hospital, as the old one, built in 1804, did not live up to the required standards and was much too small for the growing Jewish population. Maurycy Lazarus (1832–1912), long-term director of the Galician Mortgage Bank[1] (fig. 2.1) had also been chairman of the Jewish Hospital Council.[2] He understood the depth of this need and had a vision of a modern hospital of European standard.

He declared that he would build the hospital for one hundred beds using his own funds and "on February 15, 1898, in the jubilee year of the 50th anniversary of the reign of the Emperor [Franz Joseph I], he starts the construction."[3] Together with the experts he visited the leading European medical institutions to learn about the important details required

---

[*] I wish to thank Dr. Eleonora Bergman of the Emanuel Ringelblum Jewish Historical Institute in Warsaw (retired), Dr. Andrew Zalewski, former vice president of Gesher Galicia, and Sławka Kosińska for their invaluable comments during work on this chapter. I am grateful for the generosity of Dr. Irvin Lukežić, professor at the Faculty of Humanities and Social Sciences, University of Rijeka, Croatia, for sharing with me his unpublished work on Maurycy Lazarus and for providing me with his two articles about Józef Lazarus, who lived and worked in Rijeka. I am indebted to Iryna Kotlobulatova for her help with local Lviv information, photos, and identification of photographers in figures 2.9, 2.15–2.17. Bronek Pytowski cleaned up some damaged photographs; Olga Stankiewicz-Nakken and Włodek Stankiewicz helped with archival material; while Piotr Biliński in Germany and Dr. Adam Górski at the Institute of History, Jagiellonian University in Kraków, Poland, were instrumental in providing translation of documents and letters in German, especially those with illegible handwriting.

[1] Imperial-Royal Privileged Joint-Stock Galician Mortgage Bank (Polish: Cesarsko-Królewski Uprzywilejowany Galicyjski Akcyjny Bank Hipoteczny).

[2] Henryk Mehrer, *Szpital lwowskiej gminy wyznaniowej izraelickiej fundacyi Maurycego Lazarusa* (Lwów: Szpital Lwowskiej Gminy Wyzn. Izraelickiej, 1906), 40.

[3] Ibid., 42. This was, in fact, the project committment date, rather than the construction start date.

in a modern hospital.[4] The construction of the hospital was entrusted to the renowned Lviv firm of Ivan Levyns'kyi, also known as Jan Lewiński. The formal inauguration of the hospital took place on June 7, 1903 (fig. 2.2). The hospital was fully equipped with the private funds of Maurycy's wife, Róża Maria (Rosa Marie) née Jolles (1838–1905). This hospital is still active today, 120 years later, as the municipal maternity hospital in Lviv.

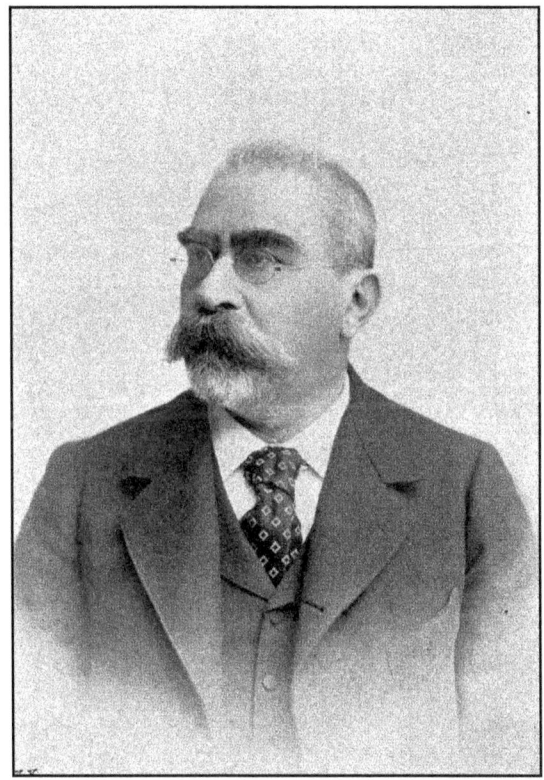

Figure 2.1. Maurycy Lazarus, photo Marek Münz, Lviv, 1903–1905. Courtesy of Iryna Kotlobulatova.

During the life of Maurycy Lazarus, Lviv was the capital of Galicia, a territory which became part of the Habsburg Monarchy after the Partition of Poland in 1772. Eastern Galicia was mainly a rural province with poor peasants largely Ruthenians (Ukrainians) and townspeople mostly Poles, Jews, and other smaller groups. In 1900, at the time the hospital construction was taking place, Lviv was a town of 159,877 inhabitants of whom 82,593 (51.56%) were Roman Catholic (mostly Poles), 44,254 (27.68%) were Jewish, and 29,337 (18.35%) were Greek Catholic (mostly Ruthenians).[5]

---

4 "Nowy szpital żydowski we Lwowie," *Kurjer lwowski*, June 8, 1903, 2.
5 Łukasz T. Sroka, *In the Light of Vienna: Jews in Lviv—Between Tradition and Modernisation (1867–1914)* (Berlin: Peter Lang, 2018), 34–35. Data for year 1900.

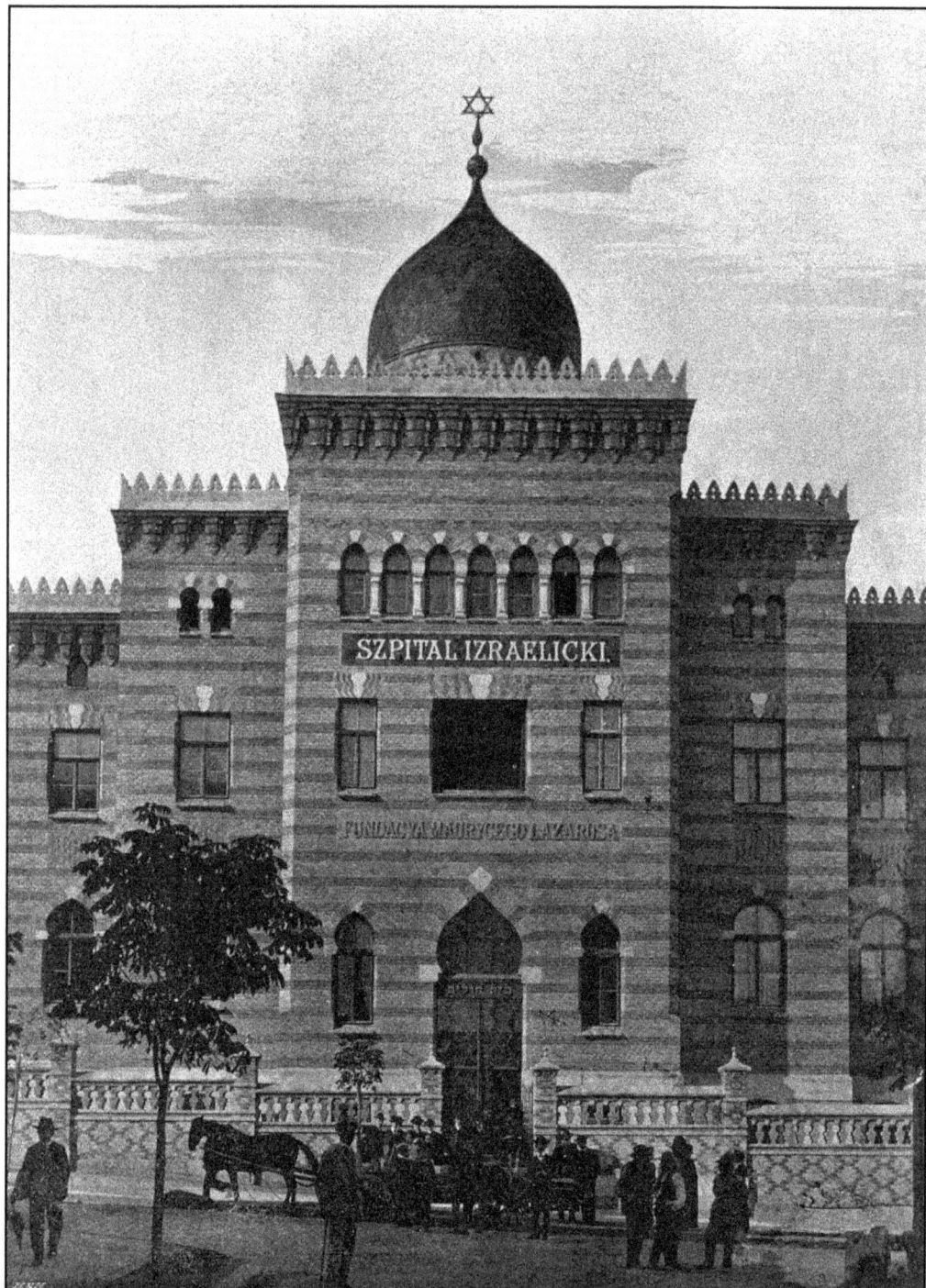

Figure 2.2. Maurycy Lazarus Foundation Israelit Hospital. Commemorative album of the city of Lviv. Publisher: Józef Pitułko. Lwów, 1904.

Maurycy Lazarus lived during a period of great social and political changes for the Jewish population of Galicia. The Habsburg Monarchy was trying to enforce the Germanization of Jews in Galicia through German-Jewish schools and by forcing them to take German last names at the end of the eighteenth century. At the same time the Haskalah (Jewish Enlightenment) movement became popular among the Jewish urban elites looking towards Vienna and Berlin.

The constitution of 1867 changed the political landscape. Even though Galician Jews were subjected mainly to German culture through the beginning of the 1880s, they began assimilating to Polish culture afterwards. An important role was played by the introduction of Polish as the official business and office language in Galicia after 1867. At the end of the nineteenth century, Lviv City Council decided to go back to the city's historical Polish street names.[6] The new city maps would show Polish names instead of the German ones that had prevailed for about a century.

At the time, several political trends coexisted in Galicia's increasingly diversified Jewish population. Large part of the Galician Jews were Orthodox, however, assimilation to Polish culture, Zionism as a response to growing antisemitism, and socialism, objecting to the poor living conditions of the urban working class, were all in play during Maurycy Lazarus's lifetime—and they involved his own family.[7]

Family history

Maurycy Lazarus was born on October 22, 1832, in Lviv. Only forty-five years earlier, in 1787, the requirement for adopting German family names had been introduced by Emperor Joseph II. It is likely that Maurycy's grandfather Lazar (1754?–1834)[8] took the surname Lazarus, using the acceptable Latinized form of the Jewish name Lazar (Hebrew: Eleazar). As tradition required, the newborn boys were given Hebrew names, which in the case of Maurycy the records show as Moses.

At the time of his birth, most Jewish families lived either in the Jewish part of the inner city, in Kraków Suburb (Krakowskie Przedmieście) or Żółkiew (Zhovkva) Suburb (Żółkiewskie Przedmieście). Figure 2.3 shows a cadastral map of the inner city of Lviv with marked birthplace of Maurycy Lazarus.

Maurycy had a sister, Rachel, born April 15, 1837, and a brother, Isaac, born August 22, 1849. He was the oldest child of Simche Lazarus (1800?–1865)[9] and Rosa née Kolischer.

---

6 Łukasz T. Sroka, *Rada Miejska we Lwowie w okresie autonomii galicyjskiej. Studium o elicie władzy* (Kraków: Wydawnictwo Naukowe Uniwersytetu Pedagogicznego, 2012), 186.
7 Information about Maurycy Lazarus and his family without a given source is largely based on stories told by members of the family born around the turn of the twentieth century (primarily Janina and Helena Diamand, granddaughters of Maurycy Lazarus) and gathered by Halina Diamand-Stankiewicz, their younger cousin.
8 Lazar Lazarus died on November 9, 1834, eighty years old. TsDIAL, fond 701, op. 1, spr. 118, f. 48, k. 642.
9 Simche Lazarus died on March 21, 1865, sixty-five years old. APP, Sign. 56/1924/0/-/19.

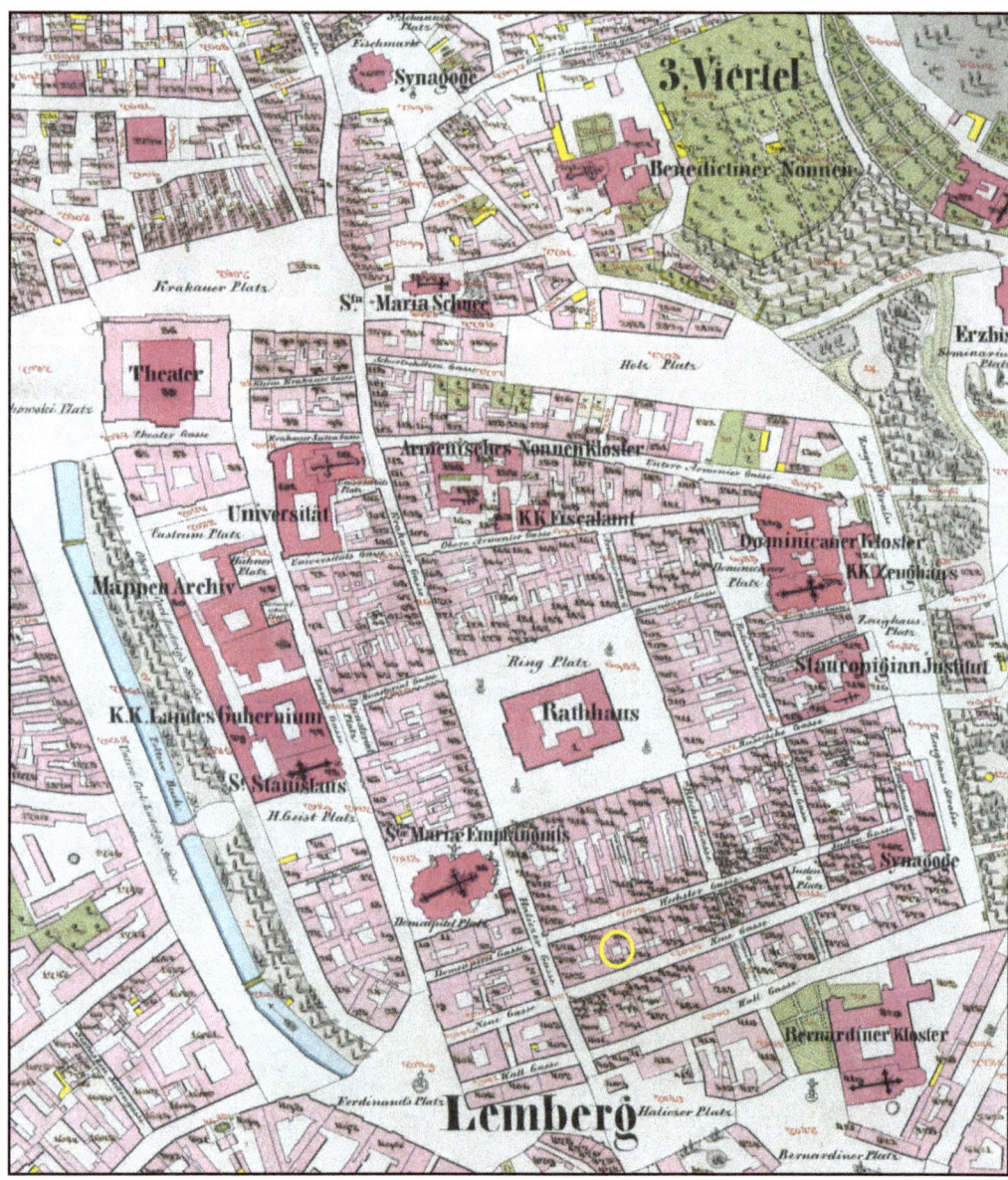

Figure 2.3. Cadastral map of the inner city of Lviv, a higly detailed graphical property records surveyed in 1849 and litographed in 1853. Original map in TsDIAL, fond 186, op. 8, spr. 628a, digital map assembly by Gesher Galicia. The cadastral map of Lviv shows the parcel numbers rather than house numbers. Jewish quarter is in the lower right portion of the map, north of the Wall Street (Wall Gasse on the map), where the city walls once were. The place where Maurycy Lazarus was born is marked with a yellow circle.

Both families had been in Lviv for generations. Simche was a wine merchant[10] and his father, Lazar, was a merchant, too.[11]

Simche and Rosa married in 1831.[12] At the time, there were several restrictions on Jewish marriages in order to limit the Jewish population in Galicia. Since 1773, it had been required for Galician Jews to obtain special permission to marry given by civilian authorities. Galicia's Jewish Edict of 1776 stated: "No Jew shall be allowed to marry unless he can prove his true merit, the permission he has received from the authorities to marry, and the taxes he has paid for this purpose." The Edict of 1785 defined the amount of the marriage tax based on family income. The marriage tax was doubled with each son wishing to wed.[13]

The Edict of Toleration (Toleranzpatent) for the Jews of Galicia from 1789 further revised requirements for Jews who wanted to marry to attend a secular German Jewish school or to have a similar education at home and pass a test. These schools were strongly opposed by the traditional Jews of Galicia. After they were closed in 1806, couples needed to pass a morality test, namely, a religious examination based on Herz Homberg's *Bne Zion: ein religiös—moralistisches Lehrbuch für die Jugend israelitischer Nation*.[14] There were additional residential restrictions for Jews in Lviv. By decree of the court registry, dated April 4, 1805, Lviv Jews could only marry someone belonging to the city's Jewish community;[15] failure to do so meant leaving the city voluntarily or risking expulsion.[16]

Few Jews applied for permission to marry and registered their traditional marriages, and most were acculturated. Orthodox Jews bypassed this process altogether and only had a ritual marriage, that is, foregoing a formal marriage record. This is a reason why large number of Jewish children were entered in birth registers as illegitimate, even if the father's name was stated. As a result, some children carried their father's name, some their mother's last name. This could cause problems later in life when proper identification was required—in the case of inheritance, for example.

In 1825 there were 44,488 Jewish families in Galicia, which increased to 46,610 families in 1826, that is, an increase of 2,122 families during that year, while there were only 137 registered marriages during this time.[17] Simche's and Rosa's marriage six years later was one of the few exceptions considered valid by secular authorities. Figure 2.4 shows their marriage permit.

---

10 LNNBU, fond 44, op. 54, spr. 92.
11 IKG, Matriken der Israelitischen Kultusgemeinde, 1784–1911.
12 TsDIAL, fond 701, op. 1, spr. 113, f. 31, k. 25.
13 Andrew Zalewski, "Jewish Marriages Revisited," *Galizianer* 28, no. 2 (2021): 10. Between 1785 and 1789 the tax was doubled for the second son and tripled for the third one. See: Majer Bałaban, *Dzieje Żydów w Galicyi i w Rzeczypospolitej Krakowskiej 1772–1868* (Lwów: Nakładem Księgarni Polskiej B. Połonieckiego, 1914), 25–27.
14 A textbook on religion and morality for the youth of the Israelite nation.
15 Małgorzata Śliż, *Galicyjscy Żydzi na drodze do równouprawnienia 1848–1914: aspekt prawny procesu emancypacji żydów w Galicji* (Kraków: Księgarnia Akademicka, 2006), 128.
16 Bałaban, *Dzieje Żydów w Galicyi*, 52–53, 73.
17 Ibid., 75. See also: Zalewski, "Jewish Marriages Revisited": 12.

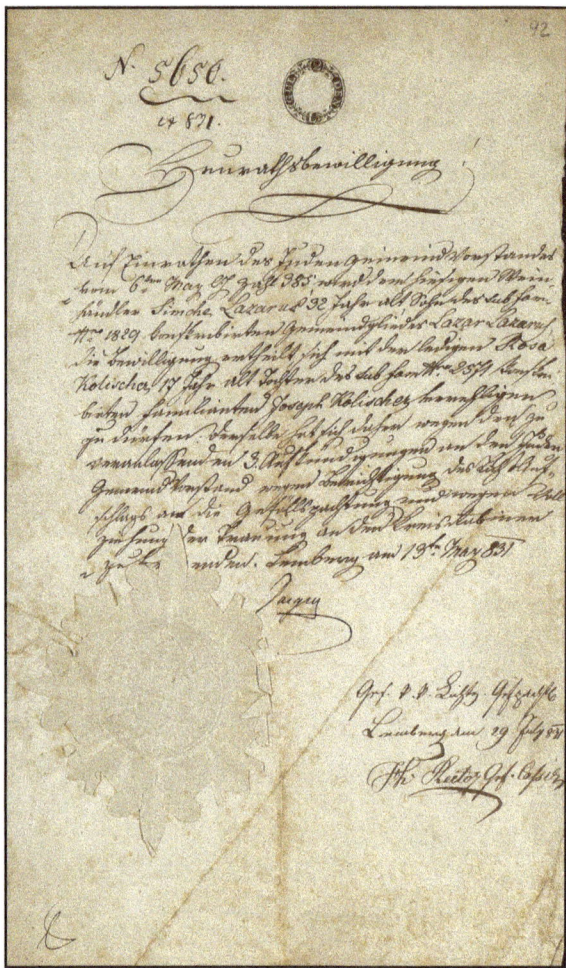

Figure 2.4. Marriage permit from 1831 for Simche Lazarus and Rosa Kolischer, parents of Maurycy Lazarus. Ossolineum, digital collection. Original in LNNBU, fond 44, op. 54, spr.92.

Due to residential restrictions, all Jewish families in Lviv at that time had a family number under which a family and all persons living in the household were registered in the family evidence books. The records were initially created during the period 1795 through 1804 and were arranged by the same congregational family numbers, as seen in the early metrical records.[18] When parents died or children married, and got their own family numbers, they were removed from the original family record. Vacated numbers were then given to a new family; this seems to have been a way to keep track of the actual number of Jewish families in town. As a consequence, Simche's family number of 987 was lower than his father's family number of 1829 or his mother's family number of 2571 (fig. 2.5).[19] However, as the original family numbers associated with a bride and a groom were shown next to their names in

---

18 Joshua Grayson, "Family Evidence Books: Another Treasure Trove," *Galitzianer* 25, no. 2 (2018): 8–9.
19 LNNBU, fond 44, op. 54, spr. 92.

the new record, it is possible to search back to previous generations. Maurycy Lazarus's grandparents, Lazar and Feige Lazarus, as well as Joseph and Mindel Kolischer, were found by searching back in time in the family evidence books.

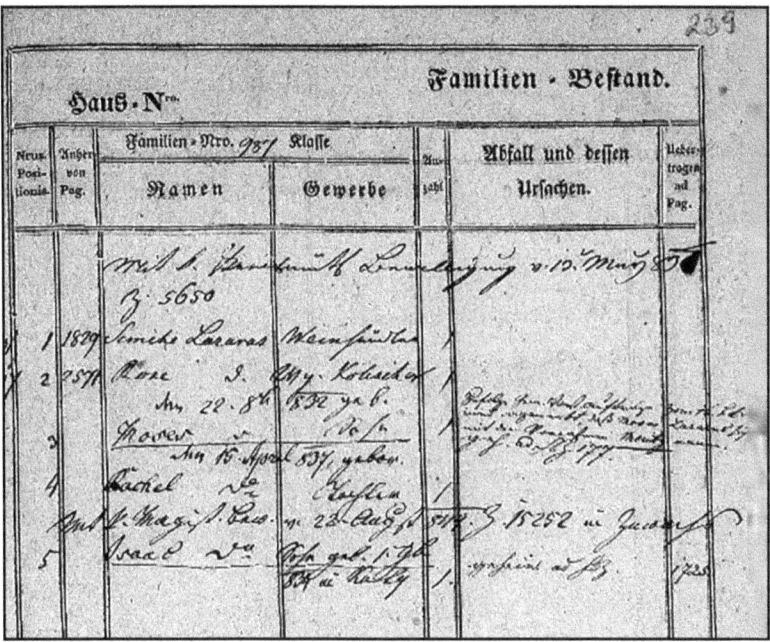

Figure 2.5. Family record for the family of Simche and Rosa Lazarus, parents of Maurycy Lazarus with the family number 987. Next to the names of Simche and Rosa are their parents' family numbers 1829 and 2571, respectively. Family Search, film #007804170, image 375. Original in TsDIAL, Lviv.

Youth

When Maurycy was of school age, there weren't any secular educational opportunities for Jewish children in Lviv. In traditional Jewish families, boys attended heder or Talmud-Torah schools (religious schools), where they learned to read and write in Hebrew, studied Torah, Talmud, and Jewish traditions, and were taught arithmetic. The lessons usually took place in the teacher's (melamed's) home, often in a very crowded setting.

The first secular schools for Jews in Galicia were opened in the early 1780s (the first school for boys in Lviv in 1782), as part of the compulsory educational system of *Normalschulen* created by Joseph II reforms for all children in the empire. The 1789 Jewish Edict of Toleration stipulated that villages and smaller towns had two-year primary schools (*Trivialschule*) and that larger towns had three-year normal schools (*Normalschule*); Lviv and Brody were required to have a four-year main school (*Hauptschule*). Herz Homberg (1749–1841), a student of Moses Mendelssohn,[20] was appointed by the emperor as the

---

20 Moses Mendelssohn (1729–1786) was the father of the Haskalah.

inspector of Jewish public schools in Galicia and mandated with creating a compulsory secular school system for Jews. Zealous in his approach, he was opposed by orthodox Jews.[21]

In 1789, when Homberg got his appointment, there were just three secular Jewish schools in Lviv: one main school and two primary schools. Under Homberg's leadership, 107 schools for boys and a few schools for girls were created in Galicia. German was the language of instruction in these so-called German-Jewish schools and there were close to four thousand pupils enrolled. However, as orthodox Jews did not trust these secular schools, they did not last beyond 1806.[22]

The next attempt to create a secular Jewish school in Lviv was not until 1842, when Maurycy was ten years old. The school was reorganized and modernized a year later, and both boys and girls could attend. It was called the Lviv German-Jewish Public Main School (Lemberger deutsch-israelitische öffentliche Hauptschule).[23] Maurycy could not have attended it, as it was established when he would have been graduating from the main school. It is most likely that he was either taught at home or attended a public Christian school and, later, a six-year public gymnasium.[24] Before 1848, there were two gymnasiums for boys in Lviv: Lviv Academic Gymnasium (Akademickie Gimnazjum Wyższe) and Lviv Gymnasium at the Dominicans (Gymnasii Leopolitani ad Dominicanos). Both taught in German at this time.[25] In addition to these, a three-years Realschule was established in 1816. In 1825, it was transformed into a school for technical sciences and trade.

In the spring of 1848, when Maurycy was fifteen and finishing his school education, Europe was burning with revolution—known as the Spring of Nations. In February 1848, the French monarchy was toppled; in the Austrian Empire, the revolution began on March 13, 1848 in Vienna; and on March 18, news about the situation in the Austrian capital reached Lviv. In both Vienna and Lviv, the citizens' National Guard was formed, which included the university students' armed Academic Legion (fig. 2.6).

A petition was sent to Emperor Ferdinand, which demanded Galician autonomy, civil liberties, national freedoms, and the abolition of serfdom.[26] Among the petitioners were Lviv's Jews. In response to the Polish demands for Galician autonomy, the Ruthenians called for national equality and a partition of the province—the eastern part Ruthenian, the western part Polish. In July 1848, both sides started a petition drive to influence the decision of the newly elected Austrian parliament. Galician Jews supported Poles in their

---

21 Mirosław Łapot, "Rozwój żydowskiego szkolnictwa świeckiego we Lwowie w latach 1772–1879," *Prace Naukowe Akademii im. Jana Długosza w Częstochowie. Pedagogika* 22 (2013): 384–385.
22 Ibid.
23 Ibid.: 386.
24 Lucyna Kudła, "Gimnazjaliści galicyjskiej doby autonomicznej. Charakterystyka społeczności," *Annales Academiae Paedagogicae Cracoviensis* 4 (2005): 98. After 1848, the length of gymnasium education was eight years. I thank Dr. Kudła for sharing with me additional information about the school system in Galicia.
25 Małgorzata Gajak-Toczek, "Męskie gimnazja państwowe we Lwowie w latach 1772–1914," *Acta Universitatis Lodziensis. Folia Litteraria Polonica* 13 (2010): 350–351.
26 Andrew Zalewski, "Soaring Hopes of 1848. Demonstrations and Petitions," *Galitzianer* 27, no. 2 (2020): 10–11.

efforts to prevent partition;²⁷ one of these was Marcus Lazarus, most likely Maurycy's uncle (fig. 2.7).²⁸

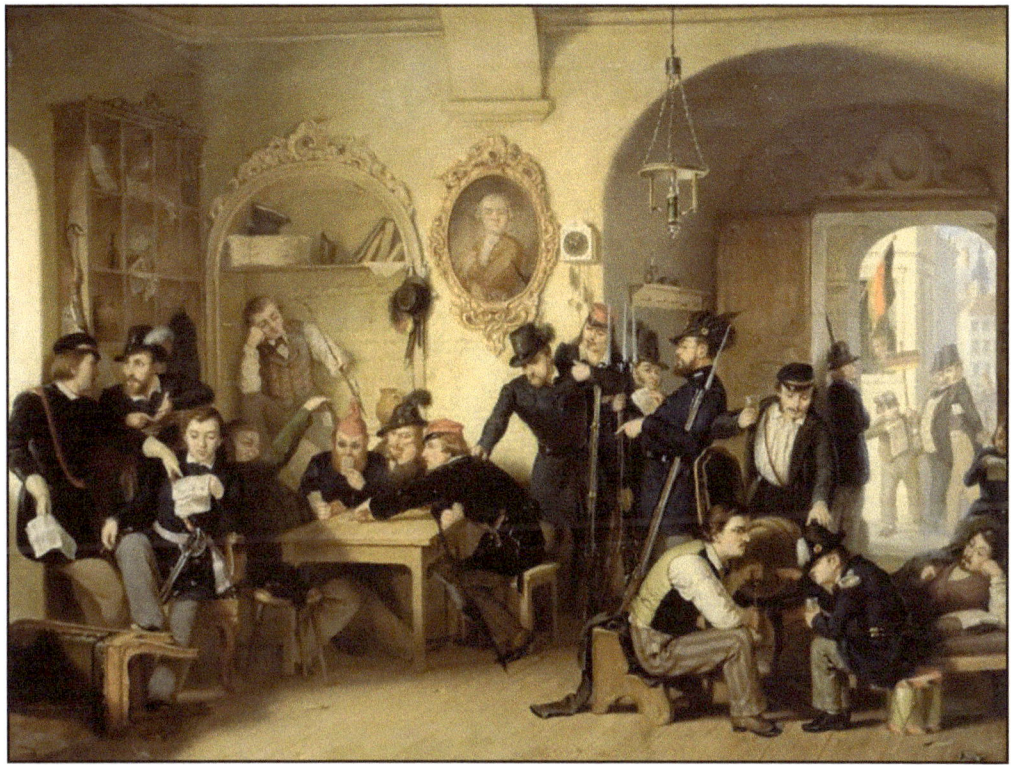

Figure 2.6. Student guard room of the Academic Legion, Vienna 1848. Franz Schams, Wien Museum, Online Collection.

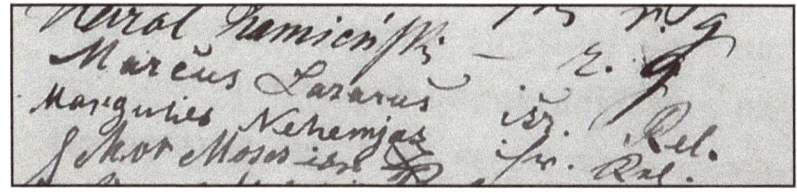

Figure 2.7. Signatures on the Petition against the partition of Galicia (July 1848). Among them is a signature of Marcus Lazarus, most likely the uncle of Maurycy Lazarus. ÖstA, HHStA LA ÖA, Series IX/130, Box 4, f. 188

At some point in 1848, Maurycy left for Vienna, where he planned to study painting, probably at the k. k. freye, vereinigte Akademie der bildenden Künste, today's Academy of Fine Arts. This is how he was later described:

---

27 Andrew Zalewski, "Jewish Petitioners. The Plan to Divide Galicia," *Galitzianer* 27, no. 4 (2020): 22–24.
28 I thank Dr. Andrew Zalewski for providing the signature of Marcus Lazarus.

Maurycy Lazarus was a spiritual child of a liberal era, a child of times when one travelled by stagecoach from Lviv to Vienna, and a faint glow of wax candles brightened the darkness of student dormitories.

The seventeen-year-old was greeted in the Danube capital by the Revolution of 1848. [...] The three-color revolution cockade with the pin is until now in the family's possession and is proof that he was on the side of the fight for freedom and social justice. Until his last days he kept this freedom cockade with reverence in his desk.[29]

By the time Maurycy arrived in Vienna, the government had closed all institutions of higher education due to the ongoing unrest. The first academic institution to reopen was the Academy of Trade. Maurycy signed up, not to waste any time. "He left the Academy prepared to become a future banker and a high-level industrialist. The knowledge he gathered would soon pave his way to the largest enterprises in Galicia and earn him millions."[30] His memories of the eventful days of 1848 remained with Maurycy Lazarus forever. In 1898 at a gathering in Vienna, he celebrated the fiftieth anniversary of the Spring of Nations with other, now graying, members of the Academic Legion.[31]

Marriage

On June 9, 1857, at the age of twenty-four, Maurycy married the eighteen-year-old Róża, the daughter of Samuel N. Jolles (1800–?) and Caroline Jolles. The Jolles family moved to Brody in order to take advantage of the commercial opportunities for which this border town—a hub of commerce in Galicia—was renowned. Later, Samuel Jolles moved his family to Leipzig, seeking prosperity there. He was not as successful in Leipzig as he had hoped, perhaps because, rather than dealing with business matters, he was more interested in reading German poets and philosophers and taking care of his canaries. He had four daughters and one son.

The wedding of Maurycy and Róża took place in Brody (fig. 2.8). The newlyweds were, according to family accounts, "religiously indifferent." When the new bride arrived in Lviv, Maurycy was advised to invite his relatives for a Shabbat dinner to please her. Traditionally, the lady of the house would say the prayer over the candles. Abashed, Róża asked her young husband what she was supposed to say. He answered that he did not know either. They agreed that she would mumble something under her breath and if there were any questions, they would explain that customs were different where she grew up. Once they got to know

---

29 At that time, he was, in fact, about sixteen years old. Henryk Feuerstein, "Lazarus: życie i czyny żydowskiego filantropa," in *Almanach Żydowski wydany przez Hermana Stachla zawierający szereg artykułów wybitnych literatów, polityków i publicystów oraz życiorysy czołowych postaci Małopolski Wschodniej* (Lwów: Wydawnictwo Kultura i Sztuka, 1937), 216. Translation E. H.
30 Ibid.
31 "Telegramy 'Kurjera lwowskiego'. Wiedeń 12 Marca." *Kurjer lwowski*, March 13, 1898, 4.

each other better, they no longer celebrated traditional holidays. The only religious rite they continued to observe was circumcision. However, when their second son died, as the result of an infection, they did not continue the custom with their youngest son.

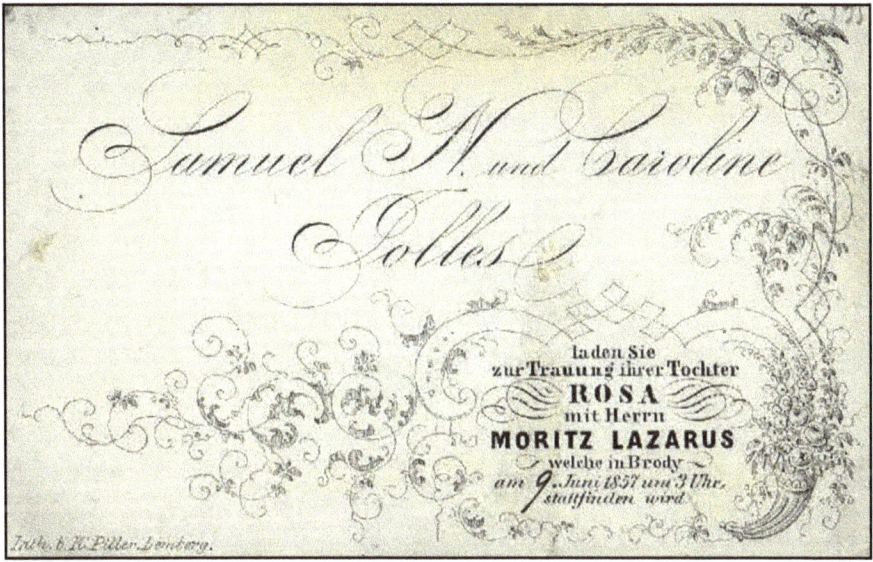

Figure 2.8. Wedding invitation to Maurycy Lazarus and Róża Jolles wedding. Ossolineum, digital collection. Original in LNNBU, fond 44, op. 40, spr. 195.

The banker

The early professional life of Maurycy Lazarus is not well known. There was a vague memory among family members that he got some banking experience, most likely in Chernivtsi (Czerniowce). Two other sources mention his early business experiences. The first is a passage in a book by Marian Rosco-Bogdanowicz, chamberlain at the court of Emperor Franz Joseph I:

> [Lazarus] was a strange personality. This respectable and good-hearted Lviv Jew started his life career with a hat store in the Andreolli passage. He ended up as the rich and omnipotent director of the Galician Mortgage Bank and an influential member of the supervisory boards of almost all major Lviv financial institutions. From under his bushy eyebrows was a menacing look that strangely softened when our benevolent ladies appealed to his pockets for charity. He made and left a large fortune thanks to his work and foresight and—a rare occurrence in such cases—I never heard of any accusation being made against him.[32]

---

32 Marian Rosco-Bogdanowicz, *Wspomnienia*, part 2 (Kraków: Wydawnictwo Literackie, 1959). Translation EH.

The second mention is in his obituary (1912): "After graduating from the university, he devoted himself to the commercial profession and as the manager of a Lviv factory he gave the first impulse to the industrialization of Galicia."[33] However, Maurycy was a banker for most of his life.

The Galician Mortgage Bank was established in Lviv on July 16, 1867.[34] It was the first joint-stock bank in Galicia. Thanks to political liberalization, eight banks were created in Galicia between 1867 and 1873, of which only two survived until the end of the nineteenth century.[35] The Galician Mortgage Bank was one of them, and the only one out of the four original mortgage banks. As a result, the bank had no competition (except for the Galician National Bank, created in 1883) until 1910.[36]

Galician Mortgage Bank's founders were members of the Polish nobility (Włodzimierz Dzieduszycki, Stanisław Gołuchowski, Alfred Józef Potocki, and Ludwik Skrzyński) and a prominent Jew from Lviv—Józef Kolischer.[37] It was Kolischer who initiated the establishment of the bank. The institution's main offices were located at 15 Halytska Square (Plac Halicki 15) in center of Lviv (fig. 2.9). Maurycy Lazarus became one of the original directors of the bank and was in charge of the commercial division. He stayed in this position for nearly four decades (fig. 2.10).

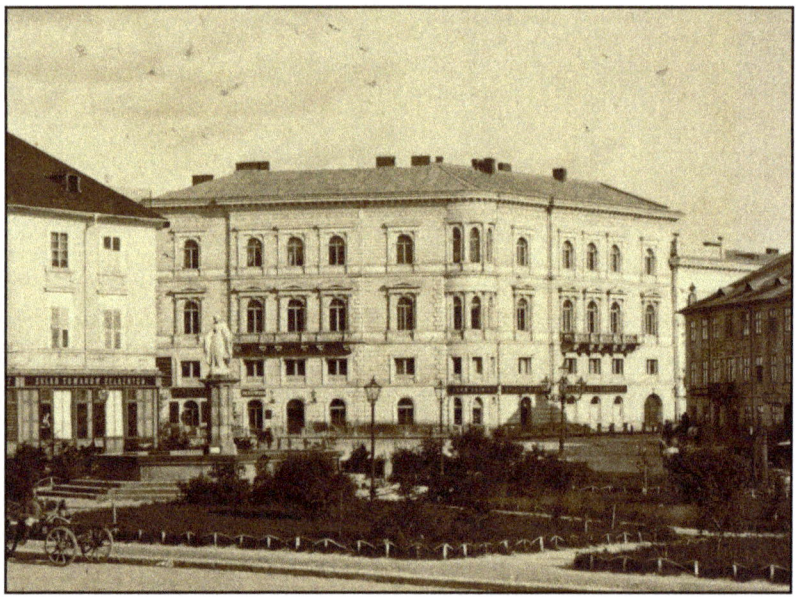

Figure 2.9. Galician Mortgage Bank built 1874. Photo: Józef Eder, 1874–1880. From the Kotlobulatovy family collection.

---

33 "Lemberg," *Die Wahrheit*, May 3, 1912, 8.
34 *Statuta c.k. uprzyw. galicyjskiego akcyjnego Banku hipotecznego* (Lwów: Drukiem Kornela Pillera, 1867).
35 Janusz Kaliński, "Bankowość austriacka na ziemiach polskich," in *Między stabilizacją a ekspansją. System Finansowy w służbie modernizacji*, ed. J. Łazor and W. Morawski (Gajt Wydawnictwo S. C., 2014), 269, 270.
36 Wojciech Morawski, "Akcyjny Bank Hipoteczny SA we Lwowie," in *Słownik Historyczny Bankowości Polskiej do 1939 roku* (Warsaw: Muza SA, 1998), 89–90.
37 *Statuta Banku hipotecznego*, 3.

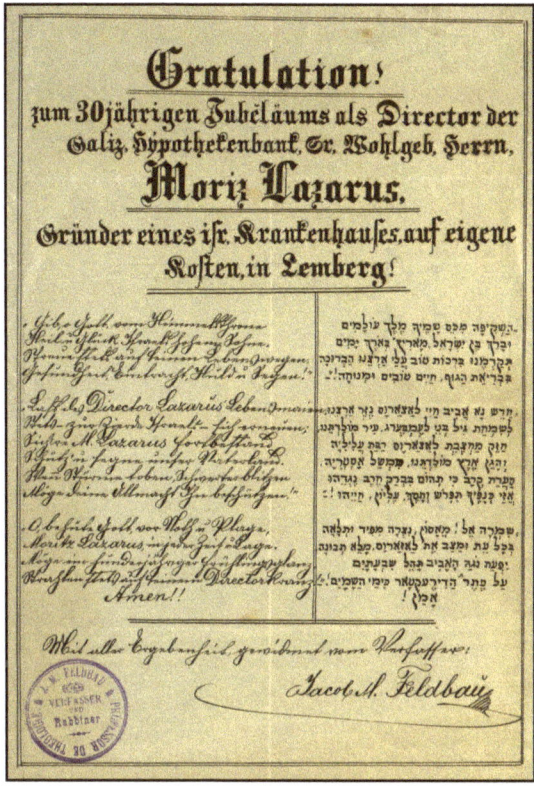

Figure 2.10. Congratulation letter for Maurycy Lazarus 30th anniversary as the Director of the Galician Mortgage Bank. Ossolineum, digital collection. Original in LNNBU, fond 44, op. 54, spr. 104.

Lazarus was also a well-respected banker in Vienna. When the Galician Credit Bank (Galicyjski Bank Kredytowy) got into trouble in 1899 and there was a run on the bank, the Polish aristocrats who comprised the board provided eight million from their own funds to cover the required sum. The already mentioned Marian Rosco-Bogdanowicz wrote:

> In addition to the cash the bank could dispose of, there was a shortfall of 1,600,000 for this purpose. A short-term promissory note loan was sought from the Wiener Bank-Verein. The signatures of Princes Adam and Władysław Sapieha, Prince Eustachy Sanguszko, both Badenis and Count Mieczysław Borkowski were offered. Bank-Verein demanded a seventh—Director Lazarus of the Mortgage Bank. How humiliating. The promissory note issued by six great and wealthy Polish aristocrats became full value only when a seventh signature—a Jewish one—was placed next to theirs.[38]

As a result of his position in the banking world, Maurycy Lazarus became a member of the board of directors of the railroad that linked Lviv and Yavoriv (Jaworów). His involvement in this project resulted in the town of Yavoriv bestowing the title of honorary citizen on him.

---

38 Marian Rosco-Bogdanowicz, *Wspomnienia*. Translation EH.

The landowner and estate owner

The Lazarus family belonged to the rising class of Jewish estate owners; wealthy Jews, who during 1866–1885 made significant investments in land and estates. Among them were the Jewish pioneers of Polonization.[39] Maurycy Lazarus bought one such property at an auction in around 1880. A couple of years later, together with Samuel Horowitz and Szymon Schaff, whom he brought in as co-owners,[40] he created a large timber company registered as State of Brody (Państwo Brody), with offices in Lviv. He also owned property in Czarna, close to Ustrzyki Dolne, where the local post office was listed in his name[41] and was the owner of property in Grabownica (fig. 2.11), near the small town of Nowe Miasto (now Nove Misto, Ukraine). He had other incorporated properties as well.[42]

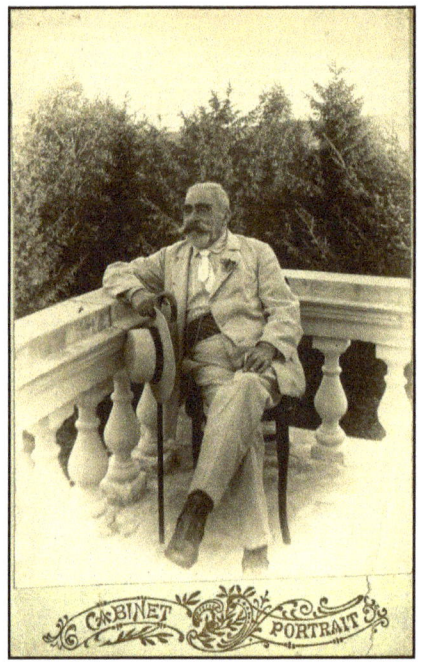

Figure 2.11. Maurycy Lazarus in Grabownica August 30, 1907. Ossolineum, digital collection. Original in LNNBU, fond 44, op. 61, spr. 32.

---

39 N. M. Gelber, ed., *The Encyclopedia of the Jewish Diaspora, Poland Series: Lwów Volume (Lviv, Ukraine)*, part 1, History of the Jews of Lwów, trans. Myra Yael Ecker, JewishGen, 305–6, accessed August 14, 2023, https://www.jewishgen.org/Yizkor/lviv/lvi303.html: "Families Horowitz, Kolischer, Mises, Löwenherz, Parnas, Lazarus, Baczes, Landesberger, Dubs, Wahl, Buber, Kellermann, Rosmarin, Fraenkel or Frenkel, Thon, Niewelt, were among Galicia's first Jewish estates owners, and many of them had their offices at Lwów. These estate owners employed Jews also as clerks and in agricultural work."
40 "Etyka miljonerów," *Kurjer lwowski*, March 5, 1901, 4.
41 *Szematyzm Królestwa Galicyi i Lodomeryi z Wielkim Księstwem Krakowskim na rok 1892* (Lwów: Nakładem C. K. Namiestnictwa, 1892), 212. *Księga Adresowa Król. Stoł. Miasta Lwowa 1902* (Lwów: Wydawca Fr. Reichman, 1902), 331.
42 *Galicia 1891 Business Directory*, JewishGen, accessed August 14, 2023, https://www.jewishgen.org/databases/poland/galicia1891.htm.

The letterhead "Verwaltung der Moritz Lazarus'schen Herrschaft Odrau" (Administration of Moritz Lazarus's Dominion Odrau) on the stationery on which Lazarus wrote a letter to his children in 1905 indicates that he owned Castle Odrau in the Moravian-Silesian region of Austria-Hungary (fig. 2.12); and he is listed as the next to the last owner in the castle's records.[43] Family correspondence shows that members of the extended family met and spent a significant amount of time there. However, the favorite family place was Ostrów, an estate near Przemyśl, where the whole family liked to go for holidays and summer vacations.

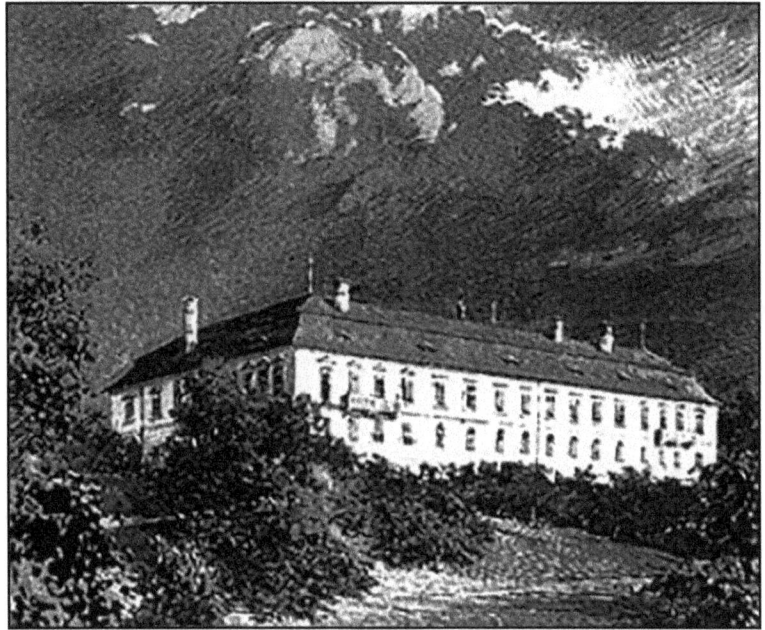

Figure 2.12. Castle Odrau in the Moravian-Silesian region of Austro-Hungary.

Political and social engagement

In December 1867, a few months after the Galician Mortgage Bank was founded, the constitution gave equal civil and political rights to all citizens of the Cisleithanian part of the dual Austro-Hungarian Empire. Emancipation opened up new opportunities for Galicia's Jews. The province received autonomy and Polish became the official tongue. Slowly, Polish language and culture started to replace German among the Jewish elite—especially among the younger generation, educated in Polish secondary schools and universities.

In 1868, the statutes of the Galician cities had yet to be decided by the Galician Sejm (National Galician Parliament; Polish: Sejm Krajowy), where there were attempts to delay equal rights for Jews. In October 1868, Lviv's statute was finally adopted and approved by

---

43 "Schloß Odrau, 700 Jahre Herrschaftssitz," Alte Heimat, Chronicle v. Rolleder, last modified September, 15, 2009, https://www.kuhlaendchen.de/media/bilder/hk-odrau/SchlossOdrau.pdf, 1–2.

the emperor. As a result, Lviv City Council removed most limitations pertaining to Jews from its statute. The involvement of Maurycy Lazarus in community affairs was soon visible at city level. He took part in the 1871 and 1877 elections to city council from the second electoral curia (voting block), representing Lviv's chamber of commerce and industry,[44] and received an overwhelming majority of electoral votes (fig. 2.13).[45]

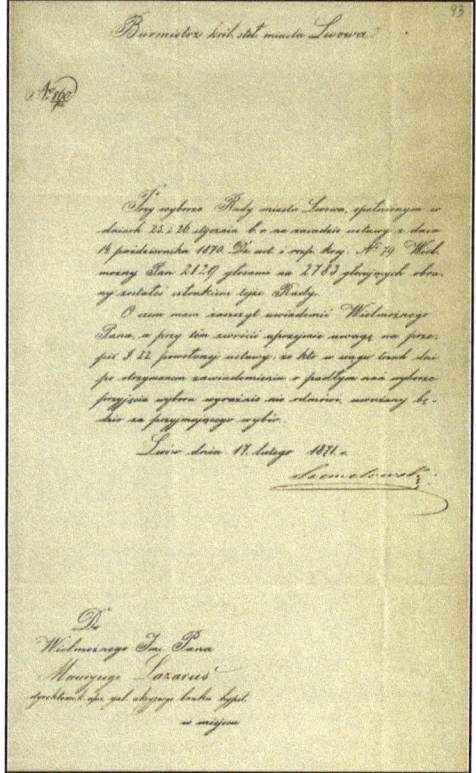 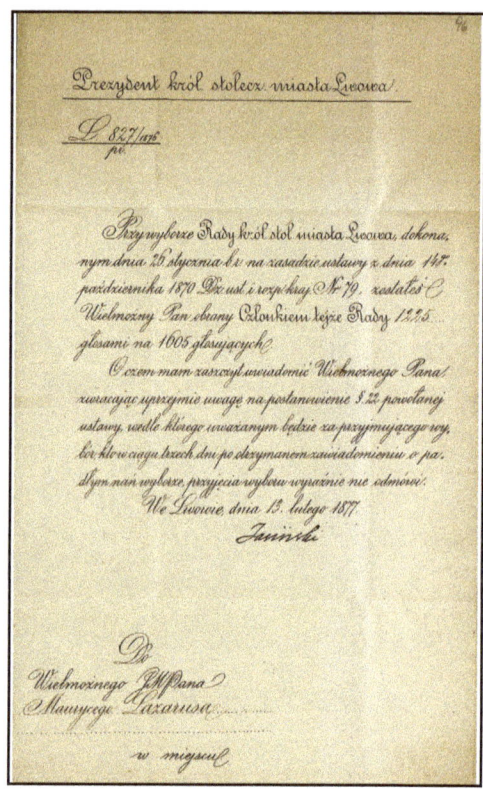

Figure 2.13. Letters informing Maurycy Lazarus about him winning the elections to the Lviv City Council in 1871 (left) and 1877 (right). Ossolineum, digital collection. Original in LNNBU, fond 44, op.54, spr. 93 and 96.

In October 1876, he was also elected to the Galician Sejm (fig. 2.14), which had been created fifteen years earlier. Initially, the first elections in 1861 were planned without Jewish participation, which outraged the province's Jews. A delegation of Galician Jews went to Vienna to fight for Jewish rights, and in a March 1, 1861 decree, the emperor granted them

---

44 There were also the Kraków and Brody chambers of commerce. Lviv's chamber of commerce covered the region with the largest population of 2.4 million people.
45 In the 1871 election, Maurycy Lazarus received 2,129 votes out of 2,783 (LNNBU, fond 44, rkps 54, spr. 93); in the 1877 election, he received 1,225 votes out of 1,605 (LNNBU, fond 44, rkps 54, spr. 96). Second electoral curia had indirect elections, so in reality the vote in 1871 represented 32,654 merchants and industrialists from thirty districts (data from the end of 1870). See: *Szematyzm królestwa Galicyi i Lodomeryi z wielkiem księstwem krakowskiem na rok 1872* (Lwów: z drukarni E. Winiarza, 1872), 303.

active and passive voting rights.[46] Although Maurycy Lazarus was elected to the Galician Sejm for the period 1877–1882, he gave up his mandate in September 1878. This was probably because he lost the election to the board of the chamber of commerce, even though it was not necessary to be a member of the board in order to represent the chamber in the Galician Sejm.[47]

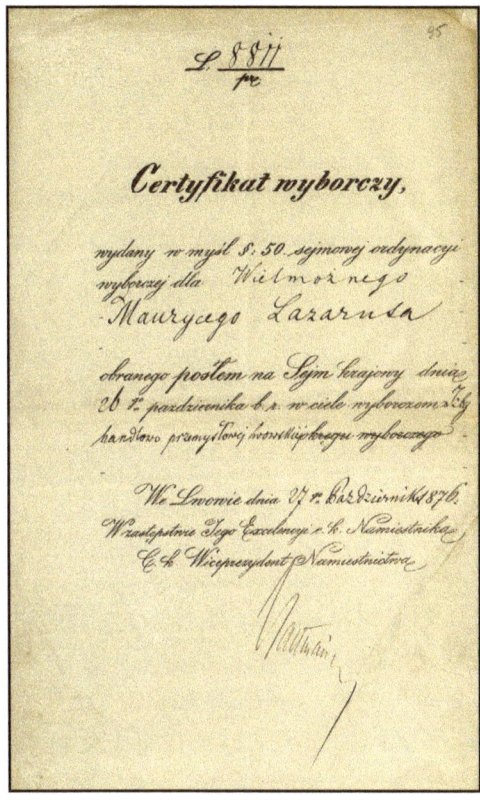

Figure 2.14. Election Certificate for Maurycy Lazarus winning the election to the Galician Sejm. Ossolineum, digital collection. Original in LNNBU, fond 44, op.54, spr. 95.

When the Society of Progressive Jews "Shomer Israel" (Guardian of Israel) and its publication *Der Israelit* was formed in 1868 in Lviv, Maurycy Lazarus was, together with other prominent Jews, a member of the organizing committee. At the time, the Jewish upper class was still leaning towards German culture and Viennese liberal-intellectual spheres. Those tendencies were contrary to the politics of the Polish majority in Galicia, which was trying to gain the maximum possible autonomy. "Shomer Israel" members feared that too much dependence on the Polish elites would negatively

---

46 Bałaban, *Dzieje Żydów w Galicyi*, 193.
47 *Gazeta Lwowska*, no 233, September 20, 1878, 2; Konrad Meus, *Izba Handlowa i Przemysłowa we Lwowie (1850–1918) Instytucja: i ludzie* (Kraków: Wydawnictwo Naukowe Instytutu Pedagogicznego, 2021), 98–99.

impact Jews.[48] According to Majer Bałaban, "Shomer Israel was born one generation too late, although in fact before that, i.e., before the constitution, it could not have been born, as in the absolute state there was no place for political associations at all, much less for Jewish ones."[49]

After receiving recognition as a political organization in 1873, "Shomer Israel" took part in the first direct elections to the Reichsrat (pan-Austrian parliament), creating the first Jewish electoral committee (Central-Wahlcomité der Juden in Galizien). It ran against the politically conservative Polish bloc and in alliance with Ruthenian Council (Ruska Rada). The chairman of the electoral committee was Juliusz Kolischer, the vice chairmen, Maurycy Lazarus and Józef Kohn. The alliance won three urban seats, and Herman Mieses, Joachim Landau, and Oswald Honigsmann took seats in parliament.[50]

The Polish distrust of Jews caused by the 1873 elections lasted a long time. In the years to follow, "Shomer Israel" concentrated its efforts on activities within the Jewish community, especially those concerned with local leadership, where they were able to win seats on the Lviv Jewish Community Council. They also won seats on the Lviv City Council.[51] But times were changing. In the 1879 elections to the Austrian parliament, "Shomer Israel" aligned itself with the Poles under the leadership of Emil Byk, who "took the view that the Jews' interest was best served by joining the Poles."[52]

In 1880, Maurycy Lazarus gave up his position on the Jewish Community Council to become the chairman of the Jewish Hospital Council in Lviv, a position he held until his death.[53] During his time on the council, he would observe the shortcomings of the old hospital, founded in 1804, and its inability to serve the growing Jewish population of the city. A dream of a modern facility that adhered to the highest European standards gradually took shape. In the meantime, however, he was busy with other initiatives and his business activities as the director of the Galician Mortgage Bank.

In 1888, Baron Maurice de Hirsch (1831–1896), a great German-born Jewish philanthropist living in Paris and creator of the Ottoman Empire's railroad system, as well as the first railroad from Paris to Constantinople (Istanbul), a line best known for the *Orient Express*, pledged twelve million francs towards the creation of an Austria

---

48 "Szomer Israel we Lwowie," Muzeum Historii Żydów Polskich POLIN, accessed April 29, 2023, https://sztetl.org.pl/pl/miejscowosci/l/703-lwow/101-organizacje-i-instytucje-spoleczne/81036-szomer-israel-we-lwowie.
49 Majer Bałaban, *Historia lwowskiej synagogi postępowej* (Lwów: Zarząd Synagogi Postępowej we Lwowie, 1937), 121.
50 Rachel Manekin, "Politics, Religion and National Identity: The Galician Jewish Vote in the 1873 Parliamentary Elections," in *Focusing on Galicia: Jews, Poles and Ukrainians 1772–1918*. Polin. Studies in Polish Jewry, vol. 12, ed. Israel Bartal and Antony Polonsky (Oxford: The Littman Library of Jewish Civilization, 1999), 105, 117.
51 Rachel Manekin, "Shomer Yisra'el," YIVO Encyclopedia of Jews in Eastern Europe, accessed March 22, 2023, https://yivoencyclopedia.org/article.aspx/Shomer_Yisrael.
52 N. M. Gelber, ed., *The Encyclopedia of the Jewish Diaspora, Poland*, JewishGen, 317–318, accessed March 22, 2023, https://www.jewishgen.org/Yizkor/lviv/lvi303.html.
53 Mehrer, *Szpital lwowskiej gminy*, 40. According to a family story, at some point, due to intrigues in the hospital council, an embittered Maurycy Lazarus stepped down. However, it must have been in the last year of his life, as he was still listed as its chairman in 1912, the year of his death. See: *Szematyzm Królestwa Galicyi i Lodomeryi z Wielkim Księstwem Krakowskiem na rok 1912* (Lwów: Nakładem Prezydyum C. K. Namiestnictwa, 1912), 1060.

foundation in honor of Franz Joseph I's forty-year reign. The foundation was to support impoverished Jews in Galicia and Bukovina by providing education and vocational training. The goal was to open elementary, vocational, and farming schools to prepare poor Jewish children for work in manual trades and agriculture, areas with very low Jewish participation.[54]

Maurycy Lazarus had already written on the subject in 1885 in a book titled *Juden als Ackerbauern* (Jews as Farmers).[55] He was one of the people consulted about the needs of the Galician Jews by Baron Hirsch's representative during his visit to Galicia in September 1889 to speed up the creation of the foundation. Unfortunately, due to local resistance, the process was significantly delayed.[56] Finally, "Agudas Achim" (the "Covenant of Brothers" Society) prompted the Speaker of the Galician Sejm to convene a survey in May of 1890.[57]

A delegation was also dispatched to Vienna composed of Samuel Horowitz, president of the Jewish Community, Maurycy Lazarus, and Jakub Piepes, president of "Agudas Achim", which indirectly helped to achieve the agreement between the government and the founder.[58] The foundation board was formed in Vienna and three executive committees were installed in Kraków, Lviv, and Chernivtsi. Maurycy Lazarus became president of the executive committee in Lviv, established on May 21, 1891.[59] He was also president of the Lviv branch of the Israelite Alliance of Vienna (Israelitische Allianz zu Wien),[60] a charitable organization founded in 1872. From 1892, the alliance pursued its educational work in Galicia through the Baron de Hirsch Foundation.[61]

Maurycy Lazarus participated in a wide range of projects which addressed the needs of both his Jewish compatriots and his city. When the General Regional Exhibition was held in Lviv in 1894 (fig. 2.15), on the centenary of the Kościuszko Uprising against tsarist Russia, he was a member of the organizing committee. This was a Galician exhibition showcasing the whole province and the successes of political autonomy. In just four months, it brought over one million visitors to a city with a population of slightly over one hundred thousand.[62] From 1870 onwards, when Lviv received its

---

54 Solomon Spitzer, *Maurycy Baron Hirsch i jego działalność filantropijna* (Kraków: Drukiem Józefa Fischera, 1891), 34–35; Matthias B. Lehman, *The Baron: Maurice de Hirsch and the Jewish nineteenth century* (Stanford: Stanford University Press, 2022), 223.
55 Moritz Lazarus, *Juden als Ackerbauern: ein Beitrag zur Lösung der sozialen Frage der Juden in Galizien* (Lemberg: n.p., 1885).
56 Spitzer, *Maurycy Baron Hirsch*, 37, 39–40.
57 Polish: Towarzystwo "Przymierze Braci"—organization created in Lviv in 1882 promoting Polish acculturation. It published the bimonthly newspaper *Ojczyzna* (Fatherland) in Polish with a Hebrew supplement. See also: Spitzer, *Maurycy Baron Hirsch*, 43–44.
58 Ibid., 44.
59 Ibid., 51.
60 *Księga adresowa Król. Stoł. Miasta Lwowa* 1894, 87 and 1897, 212. "Z działalności wiedeńskiej 'Allianz' dla Galicyi," *Jedność*, May 20, 1910, 5.
61 Gotthard Deutsch and A. Kaminka, "Israelitische Allianz zu Wien," Jewish Encyclopedia, accessed April 15, 2023, https://jewishencyclopedia.com/articles/8306-israelitische-allianz-zu-wien.
62 "The General Regional Exhibition of Galicia," Center for Urban History, Lviv, accessed July 23, 2023, https://lia.lvivcenter.org/en/storymaps/exhibition-after/. "The Pavilions of the Galician General

self-governing municipal statutes, the city developed tremendously and wanted to show it. The exhibition was held in Stryiskyi Park (Park Stryjski), with a great view of the city and its surroundings (fig. 2.16), and boasted thirty-four themes, each with its own organizing committee and separate judges. A special brochure about Lviv and the exhibition was printed by the Society for the Development and Beautification of the City, of which Maurycy Lazarus was a member.[63] His timber company had its own pavilion there.[64]

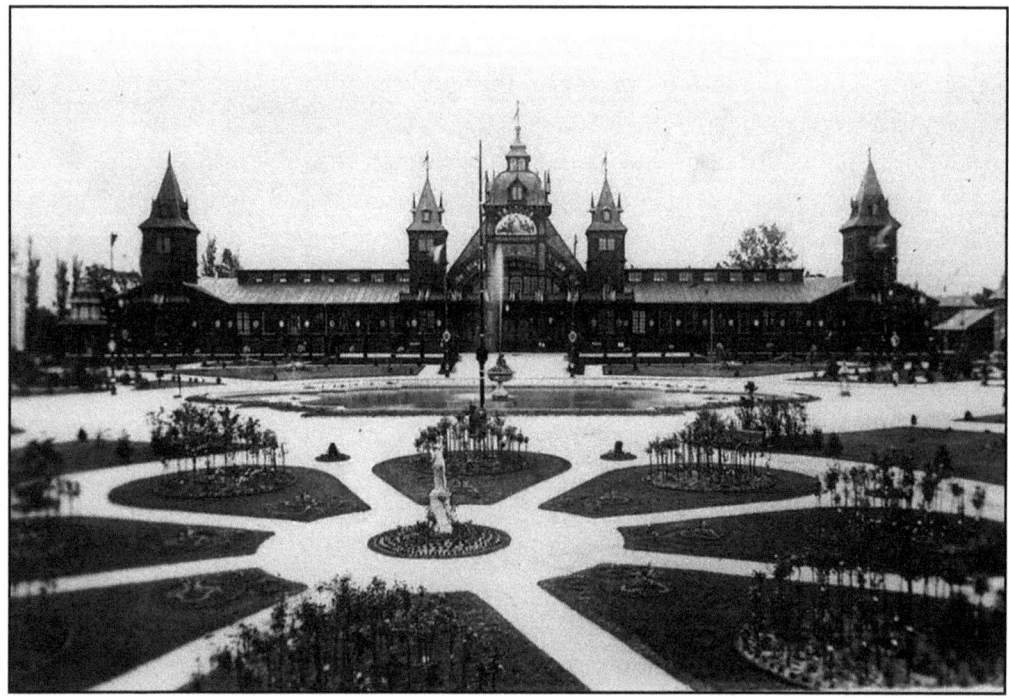

Figure 2.15. The General National Exhibition in Lviv in 1894 in Stryiskyi Park (Park Stryjski), Main Pavilion. Photo: Edward Trzemeski, 1894.

As a member of the organizing committee of the exhibition, Lazarus received a formal invitation addressed to him as "Moritz." During the planning work he was "Maurycy." He sent the invitation back, stating that he was not Moritz and if they could not accept Maurycy, they could use his Jewish name Mojżesz (Moses).[65] He used Moriz for family correspondence—mostly in German—throughout his life, however, and was addressed as

---

Regional Exhibition of 1894," Forgotten Galicia, accessed July 23, 2023, https://forgottengalicia.com/the-pavilions-of-the-galician-general-regional-exhibition-of-1894/.
63 *Ilustrowany Przewodnik po Lwowie i Powszechnej Wystawie Krajowej* (Lwów: Towarzystwo dla Rozwoju i Upiększania Miasta, 1894), insert 7.
64 Ibid., 166.
65 Feuerstein, "Lazarus: życie i czyny," 218.

such in his wife's letters.⁶⁶ This was likely because German was the language of the Jewish elites at the time they married and for years after. It could also have been because Róża grew up in Leipzig.

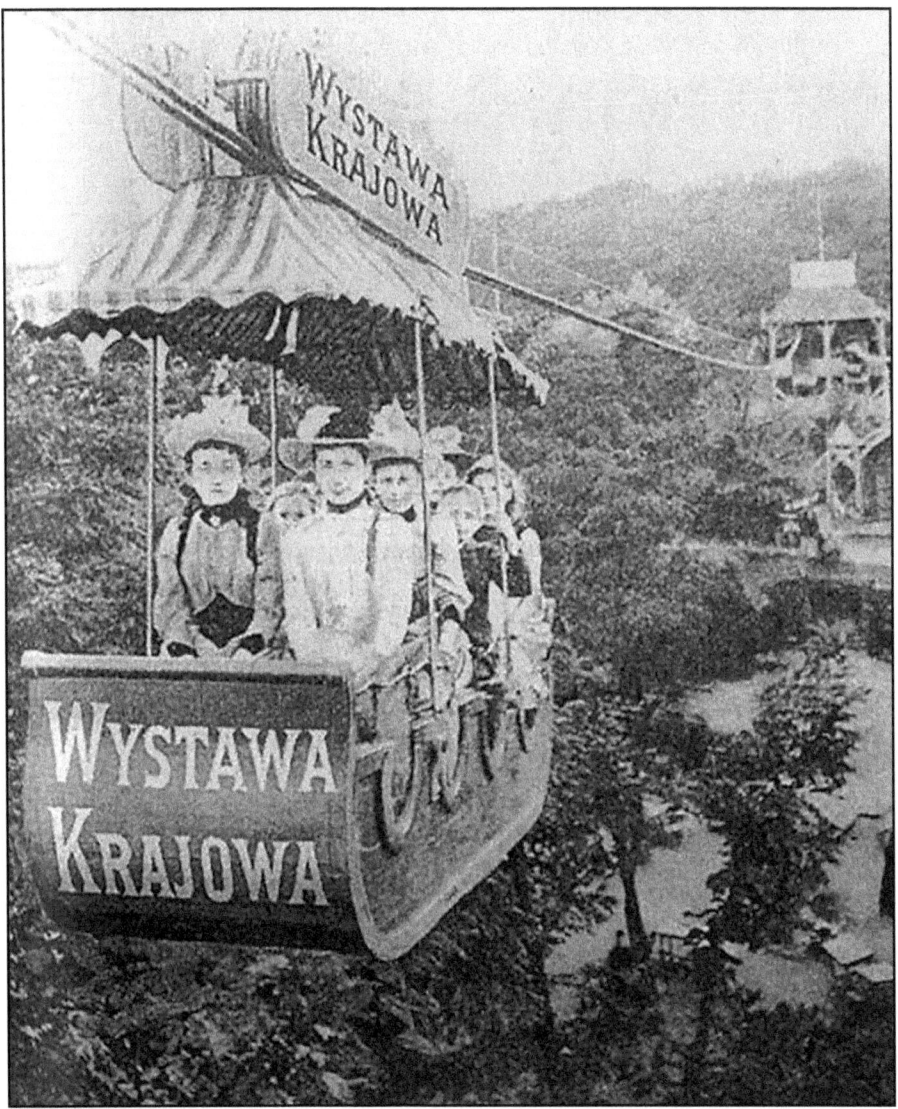

Figure 2.16. The General National Exhibition in Lviv—Aerial Tram. Photo: Edward Trzemeski, 1894.

In addition to his civic obligations Maurycy Lazarus was also deeply involved in important projects that would benefit the Jewish community. During 1894, the same year as the exhibition, a committee under his leadership was organized to finally deal with the reconstruction and repainting of the Progressive Synagogue in Lviv, known also as Tempel

---

66 Lazarus used Moritz, Moriz, and Maurycy at different points in his life or in different contexts.

(fig. 2.17)—a project to modernize the building and add a reception hall for board meetings and various festivities. The constant lack of money kept this project dormant. Architect Julian Zachariewicz, a professor at Lviv Technical University,[67] had drawn up rather grandiose plans for improvements to Tempel;[68] however, they were simply too expensive. Scaled-down plans were approved by the city in May 1896, and once the funds were available reconstruction finally started. Natan Mayer, chairman of the board of Tempel, often consulted with Maurycy Lazarus during the process.[69]

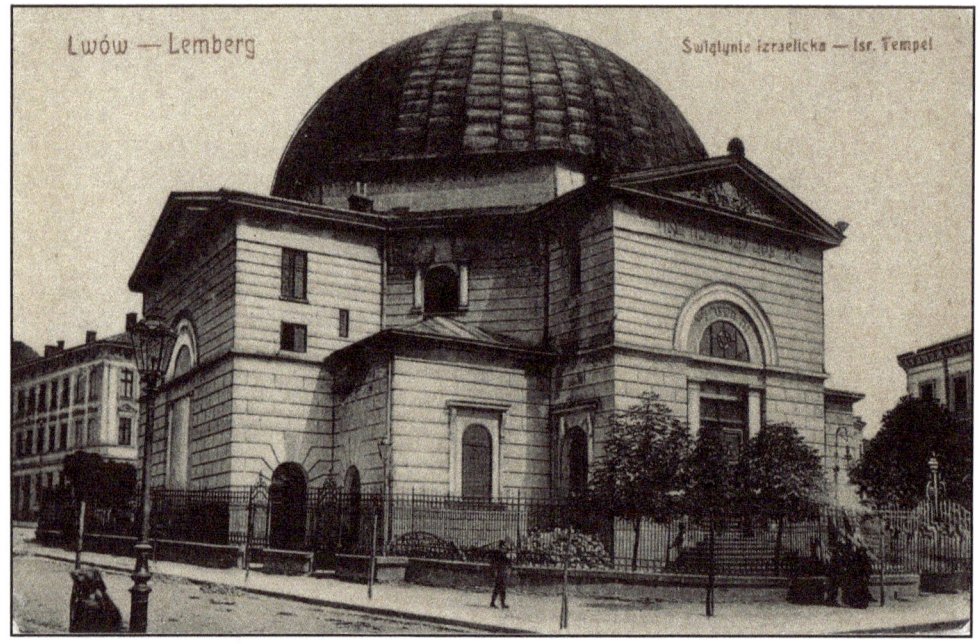

Figure 2.17. Progressive Synagogue (Tempel) in Lviv. Photo: Leopold Weis, Budapest, 1900–1908 (postcard). Courtesy of Iryna Kotlobulatova.

The philanthropist

Throughout his life Maurycy Lazarus supported humanitarian causes. The Israelite Aid Society for the Poor Jews in Galicia[70] has been listed under his name and address in the Lviv's address book over the years. He is also listed as a member of the National Association of Patriotic Aid in Galicia,[71] a section of the Austrian Red Cross which not only aided the wounded on battlefields, but also helped soldiers who were sick or invalids and widows and

---

67 For Lviv Technical University's various names over time, see footnote 48 in chapter 3.
68 Bałaban, *Historia lwowskiej synagogi*, 143–144. Bałaban describes the changes planned and points out that Zachariewicz was mistaken about the origin of the synagogues' architecture, on which he based his reconstruction plans.
69 Bałaban, *Historia lwowskiej synagogi*, 144n5.
70 Polish: Tow. izr. pomocy dla biednej ludności żydowskiej w Galicyi.
71 Polish: Krajowe Stowarzyszenie patryotycznej pomocy w Galicyi.

orphans.[72] In 1891, the association changed its name to the National Association of the Red Cross in Galicia after joining with the women's organization.[73] There is a thank you diploma to Maurycy Lazarus from Brotherly Help (Bratnia Pomoc), a student organization at Lviv Technical University, and he is mentioned in their commemorative book.[74] What stands out is his way of extending a helping hand:

> During everyday mundane work for the poorest, he usually meets with Dr. Wilhelm Holzer, an unforgettable protector of the Jewish poor in Lviv.
>
> His door stands open not only to the poor, whom he helps in both large and small matters. The help given is constructive. One person is given resources to run a workshop, another a store; still another is helped to provision a child for marriage.
>
> All this is done out of his own pocket, on his "own account." It is not only Lviv's needy Jews that turn to him. They also come from the provinces. Lazarus takes a special interest in young people with artistic aspirations. Thanks to his generous help, painters and musicians are educated. Some of them have risen to European fame. His memories of his time in Vienna have decisively influenced his appreciation and understanding of young talent.
>
> His duties as director of the bank, and participation in countless projects of a broad social nature, do not distract him for a moment from his beloved philanthropic work.[75]

When the old synagogue in a small town, Nowe Miasto, mentioned earlier, was closed for a year due to its age and the danger of collapse, and there were no funds to build a new one, local Jews sought advice from Maurycy Lazarus, whose property in Grabownica bordered the town. He decided to fund the construction of a new synagogue himself; and in March 1908, it was dedicated in the presence of the synagogue's founder and countless people from surrounding small towns.[76]

In October 1899 progressive elite Jews created Lviv's B'nei B'rith Leopolis lodge, which was dominated by intelligentsia and professionals, including several councilmen. Maurycy Lazarus was one of the original members.[77] The Independent Order of B'nei B'rith was established in New York in 1843, and its first European lodge was founded in Germany in 1880, with Austria-Hungary following soon after. The Galician branches were dependent on the grand lodge in Vienna. B'nei B'rith took inspiration from the

---

72 *Szematyzm Królestwa Galicyi i Lodomeryi z Wielkiem Ksiestwem Krakowskiem na rok 1881* (Lwów: Nakładem Galic. C. K. Namiestnictwa, 1881).
73 Ladies' National Association of Patriotic Aid of the Red Cross in Galicia (Krajowe Stowarzyszenie dam patryotycznej pomocy Czerwonego Krzyża w Galicyi).
74 *Księga Pamiątkowa Towarzystwa "Bratniej Pomocy" Słuchaczów Politechniki we Lwowie* (Lwów: Towarzystwo "Bratniej Pomocy" Słuchaczów Politechniki, 1897), 164.
75 Feuerstein, "Lazarus: życie i czyny," 217–218. Translation E. H.
76 "Nowa bożnica," *Kurjer lwowski*, April 1, 1908, 4.
77 Sroka, *Rada Miejska*, 322.

freemasonry movement, but it was limited to Jews and omitted Masonic symbolism and ritual.[78] It was mainly a humanitarian organization; its statute stated that "political, religious and community matters are excluded from the society's scope of interest."[79] The lodge had high standards and membership was considered an honor. While B'nei B'rith's charitable activities were mainly intended to help Jews, the hospital founded by Maurycy and Róża Lazarus is given as an example of humanitarian care provided also to Christians.[80]

Maurycy Lazarus was deeply involved in the planning stage of the hospital and, together with experts, visited modern European hospitals to learn about the newest technologies. In the creation of the hospital, domestic industry was used to the largest possible extent.[81] Not everyone could envision such an ambitious project, a state-of-the-art hospital with one hundred beds. There were stories about ironic comments by Samuel Horowitz (at the time president of the Lviv Jewish Community),[82] and Szymon Schaff, who looking at the detailed planning of all the hospital's functions "'advised' [Lazarus] to think about his own 'bakery' and his own 'chicken farm' for the patients in 'his' hospital."[83]

Maurycy Lazarus was held in high esteem for his many years of service as a member and chairman of the Lviv Jewish Community Council and for all his efforts on behalf of the Jewish community of Lviv. On October 8, 1902, a celebratory service was held for him at Tempel to mark his seventieth birthday.[84] "Almost all Jewish societies with their banners took part in the service."[85] A week earlier, at Tempel's Simchat Torah service, he had received a beautifully designed leather-bound letter of gratitude for his service to the Jewish community of Lviv as a member and chairman of the Jewish Community Council, a long-term chairman of the Jewish Hospital Council, the benefactor of the hospital, and for serving the community in many other ways. (fig. 2.18)[86]

---

78 Sroka, *In the Light of Vienna*, 352–353.
79 Ibid., 355.
80 Łukasz T. Sroka, "Members of the 'Leopolis' Humanitarian Society in Lvov (1899–1938): A Group Portrait," *Scripta Judaica Cracoviensia* 12 (2014): 108.
81 "Nowy szpital żydowski we Lwowie," 2.
82 Anna Jakimyszyn-Gadocha, *W trosce o zdrowie żydowskiej społeczności Lwowa (1918–1939)* (Kraków: Wydawnictwo Austeria, 2021), 57n32.
83 Feuerstein, "Lazarus: życie i czyny," 218. Translation E. H.
84 Bałaban, *Historia lwowskiej synagogi*, 184.
85 "Siedemdziesiąte urodziny," *Kurjer lwowski*, no. 296, October 25, 1902, 4.
86 Bałaban, *Historia lwowskiej synagogi*, 184n18.

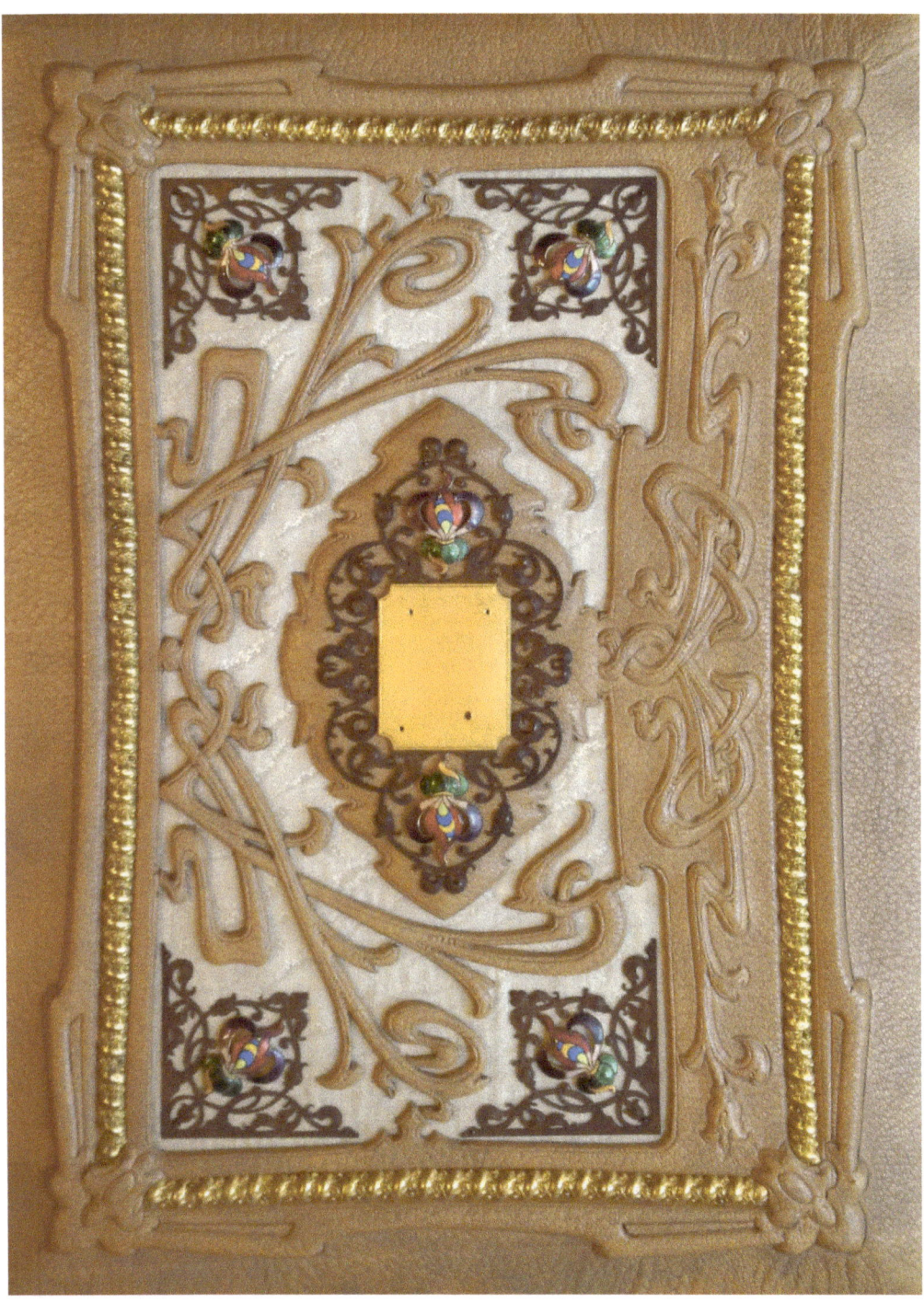

Figure 2.18 a. Leather-bound cover for the letter of gratitude presented to Maurycy Lazarus by the Jewish Community Council for his 70s birthday. LNNBU—manuscript division.

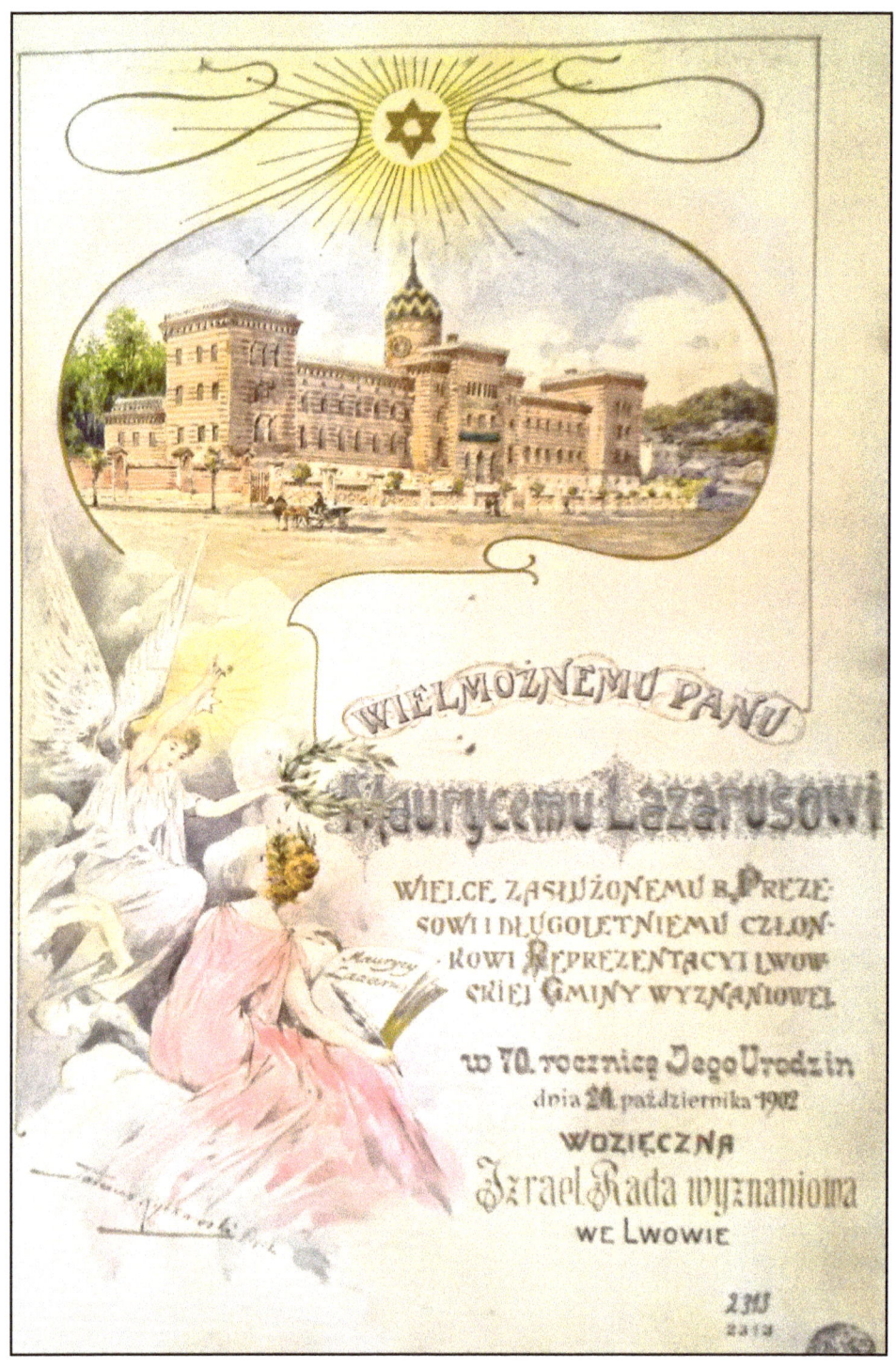

Figure 2.18 b-c. Letter of gratitude presented to Maurycy Lazarus by the Jewish Community Council for his 70s birthday. LNNBU—manuscript division.

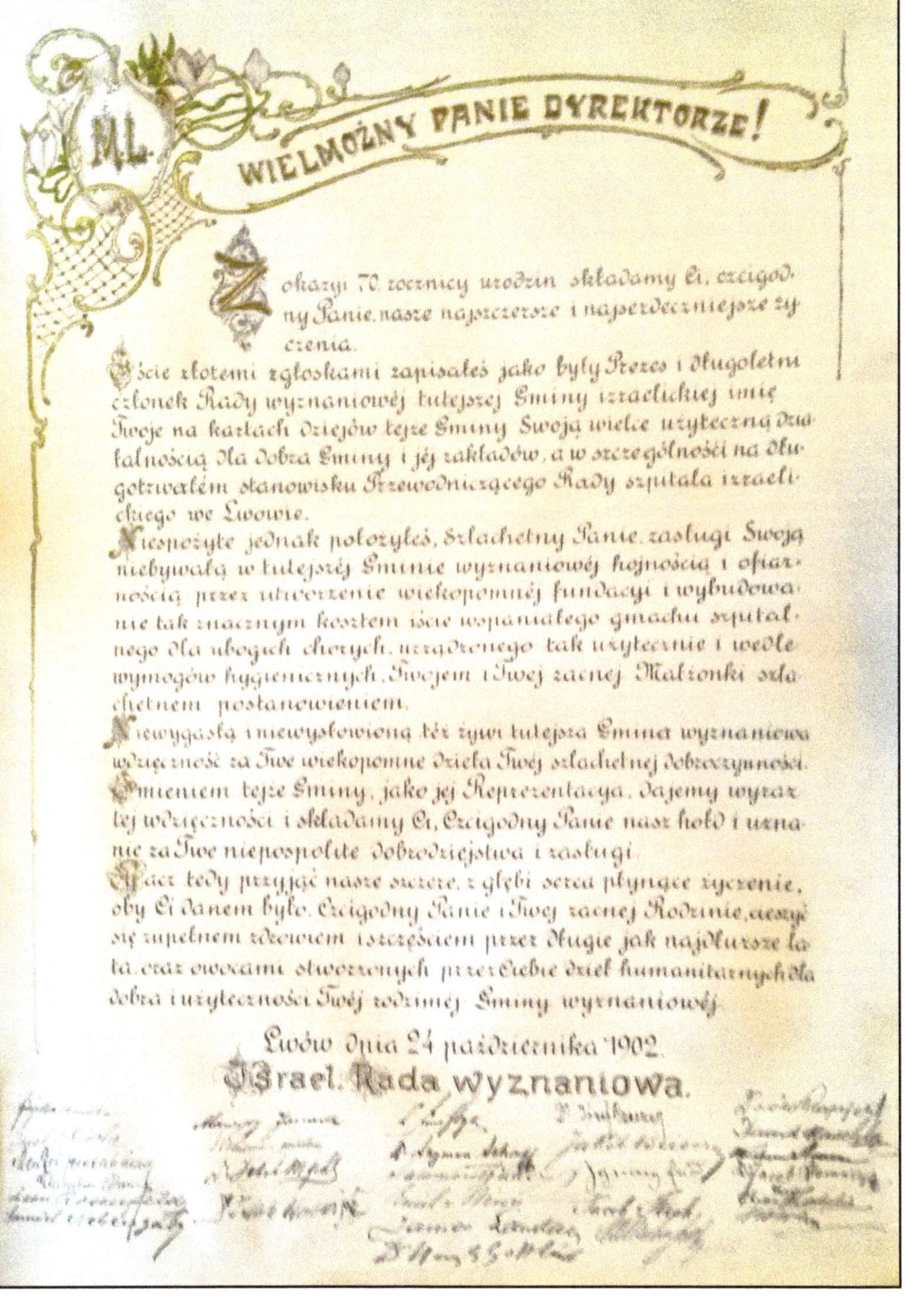

Family

The Lazarus family lived a quiet life and did not host large gatherings. This suited Róża's nature; and Maurycy satisfied with his position in society, had no need for glamour. With time, a life of comfort became one of genuine wealth. The family employed a servant, a cook, and a coachman. Having moved a couple of times, the family finally settled at 18 Słowacki (Yuliusha Slovatskoho) Street,[87] which was situated on the northeast corner of the former Jesuit Gardens (Ogród Pojezuicki), in 1919 renamed as Tadeusz Kościuszko Park; presently Ivan Franko Park.

Maurycy and Róża (fig. 2.19) had seven children.[88] There were large gaps between the children's ages and large differences in their political outlooks and ways of life.

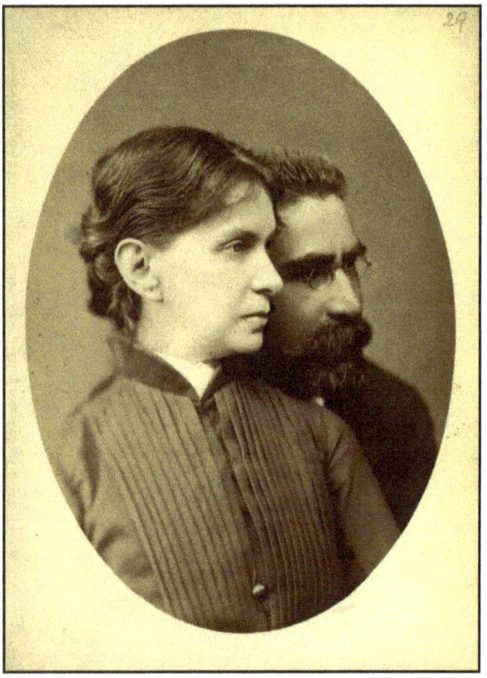

Figure 2.19. Maurycy and Róża Lazarus. Photo: Józef Eder, Lviv, circa 1880. Ossolineum, digital collection. Original in LNNBU, fond 44, op. 61, spr. 29.

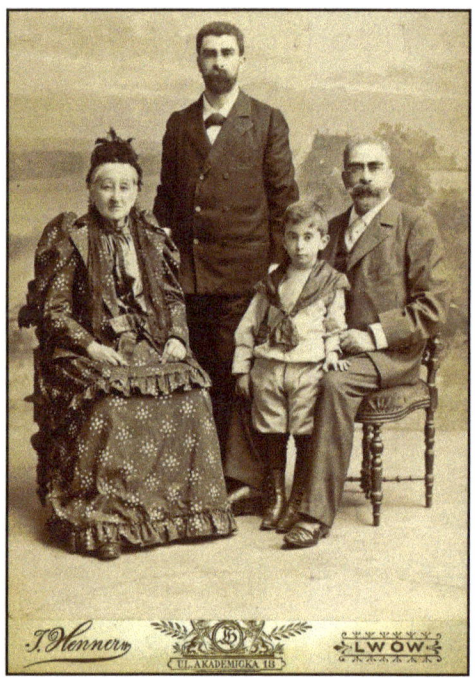

Figure 2.20. Standing - Józef Lazarus with his son Victor Karl (1888–1945). Sitting—Maurycy Lazarus and, most likely, Róża Lazarus. Photo: J. Henner, Lviv, circa 1893. Ossolineum, digital collection. Original in LNNBU, fond 44, op. 58, spr. 50.

---

87 Earlier sources show number 12, but it is the same building; the numbering has changed. I thank Iryna Kotlobulatova for this information.
88 Their oldest daughter and her mother's confidant, Wiktoria (1862–1890), died young at the age of twenty-eight and their son, born in 1865, died shortly after his birth.

Józef

The oldest son, Józef (1858–1942; fig. 2.20), studied engineering in Lviv and abroad, where he also studied shipbuilding. He became interested in religion while there, and after returning from his studies asked the Jewish Community for a mentor to help him with his religious education. The Jewish Community asked Maurycy Diamand, the father of Herman Diamand, later Józef's brother-in-law, to fulfill this role.

Józef, now Joseph, moved to Vienna, where he worked as an engineer and married Sofie Ergas (1867–1942), from a wealthy Sephardic family that originated in Ploiești, Romania. With his father's financial help, he created in 1896–1900 a shipyard in Rijeka (then Fiume), at the time part of the Kingdom of Hungary. The Viktor Lenac Shipyard, Croatia's main shipyard, was developed in 1947 on the site of the Lazarus Shipyard (fig 2.21).[89]

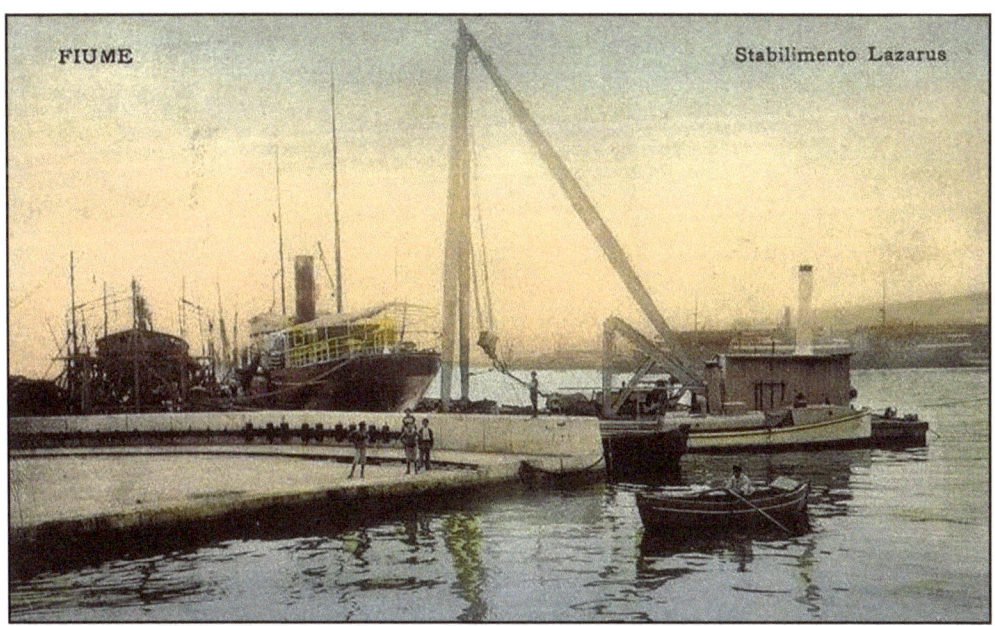

Figure 2.21. Lazarus Shipyard in 1911 on the Rijeka breakwater (postcard).

Józef (in Croatian, Josip), became active in the Jewish life in Rijeka and participated in the First and Second World Zionist Congress in Basel. He considered himself a friend of Theodor Herzl,[90] whom he may have known from Vienna, as they lived in the same district, and most likely were moving in the same circles. However, at some point after Herzl's death he left the Zionist movement. Josip Lazarus was instrumental in creating a Zionist society in Rijeka and was one of its presidents.[91] According to family stories, he retained his Polish

---

89 Irvin Lukežić, "Josip Lazarus – Prvi riječki cionist (part 2)," *Sušačka Revija* 25, no. 99–100 (2017): 33, in manuscript. I thank Dr. Lukežić for providing me with the manuscript (incl. parts 1 and 2) of his article.
90 Irvin Lukežić, "Josip Lazarus – Prvi riječki cionist (part 1)," *Sušačka Revija* 25, no. 97–98 (2017): 6, in manuscript.
91 Ibid., 18, in manuscript.

citizenship for life and was even a Polish honorary consul, something he was very proud of.[92] During his later years, he and his wife lived back in Vienna. On July 23, 1940, they fled to Zagreb.[93] Two years later, on July 9 or 10, 1942, they were captured by Ustasha forces (Croatian fascists), and on July 20, 1942 they were sent to the Jasenovac concentration and extermination camp (fig. 2.22), where they were murdered.[94]

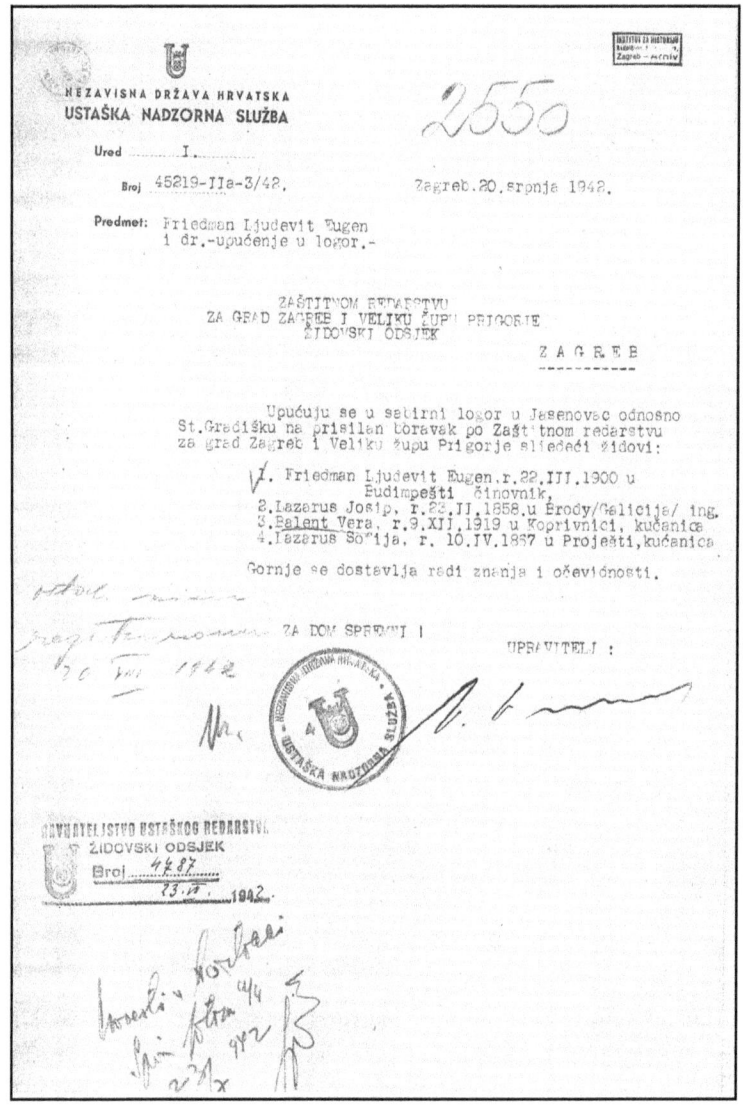

Figure 2.22. Józef and Sofie Lazarus transfer to Jasenovac concentration and extermination camp. Jasenovac Memorial Site. Original in HDA, fond 252 (RUR IURP ŽO), kut. 14, br. 29701.

---

92 This information could not be verified by the Archives of New Records (Archiwum Akt Nowych) in Poland. Most of the documents from that time were destroyed during World War II.
93 Inheritance case by Helen Lazarus, widow of Victor Lazarus, in 1957, WSTLA, WSTLA_LG_Zivilrechtssachen_A26_48T_24T_Todeserklärungen_48T_81_1957.
94 HDA, fond 252 (RUR IURP ŽO), kut. 14, br. 29701. See also: Inheritance case by Helen Lazarus in 1957 above.

Hermina, Eleonora, and Fryderyka

Three of Maurycy's and Róża's younger daughters, Hermina (1872–1951), Eleonora (1877–1944; my grandmother), and Fryderyka (1879–1942) (fig. 2.23) became involved in the socialist movement. They were educated at the private Wiktoria Niedziałkowska's eight-year gymnasium for girls, where they were introduced to socialist ideas by their teacher, Maria Wysłouch. After finishing their formal education, Hermina and a friend took additional private lessons from Mrs. Wysłouch, who read Bebel's *Die Frau und der Socialismus* (Woman and Socialism) with them. Wysłouch's influence on Hermina put her on the path to the socialist movement. She gave lectures to milliners, wrote for the socialist press using the pen name Helena Rawska, and, as Helena Rawska, she joined the Worker's Association "Strength" (fig. 2.24).[95]

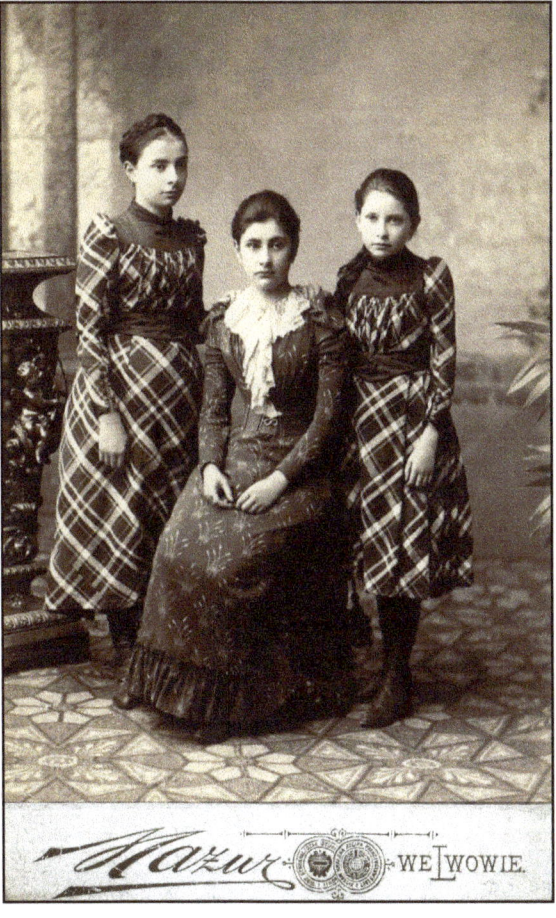

Figure 2.23. From the left: Eleonora, Hermina, and Fryderyka Lazarus. Photo: Dawid Mazur, circa 1890. Ossolineum, digital collection. Original in LNNBU, fond 44, op. 61 spr. 19.

---

95 Polish: Stowarzyszenie Robotnicze "Siła" was created in 1891; Hermina became a member in 1894 under an assumed identity, most likely to avoid her parents knowing about her activities.

In January of 1899, Hermina married Herman Diamand.[96] Her parents were strongly opposed to her union with a well-known socialist, and they tried to prevent it. After trying to secure their approval, she finally got engaged without their knowledge. Maurycy acknowledged in a communication with a family member that he did not have anything against Herman Diamand personally, but he did not want his money spent on socialist causes. Róża was probably more concerned that any scandal surrounding Hermina's decision would diminish the marriageability of her younger daughters. It seems that they were not fully aware of Hermina's own activities. Her parents made her legally renounce her inheritance, but after a few months they signed an amendment which stated that they would not enforce the document.[97] It is likely that they changed their minds when they learned that Hermina was pregnant.

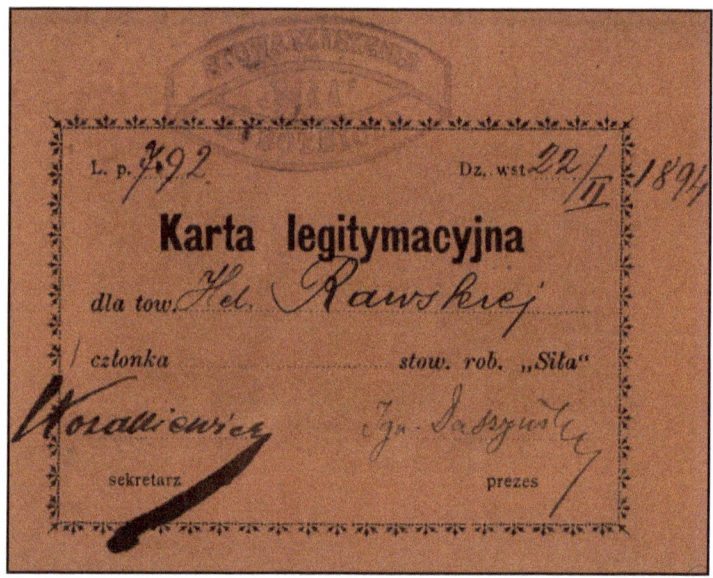

Figure 2.24. Membership card for Hermina Lazarus (assumed identity Helena Rawska) for the Worker's Association 'Strength' (Stowarzyszenie Robotnicze 'Siła'). Membership date: February 22, 1894. Ossolineum, digital collection. Original in LNNBU, fond 44, op. 42, spr. 159.

Throughout her life, Hermina was the greatest supporter and confidant of her husband, who shared with her all aspects of his political life through the more than one thousand

---

96 Herman Diamand (1860–1931) was a co-founder of the Galician Workers' Party in 1890 and the Social Democratic Party of Galicia in 1892, which became the Polish Social Democratic Party of Galicia in 1897. In 1904 he was elected a member of the International Socialist Bureau of the Second International, as a representative of Polish socialist parties in all three Partitions. After World War I he was one of the leaders of the Polish Socialist Party (PPS) and its chairman from 1928 to his death in 1931. He was a deputy to the Austrian parliament between 1907 and 1918 and to the Polish Sejm (lower house of parliament) from 1919 until 1930. He also represented Poland in several international missions in the interwar period.
97 LNNBU, fond 44, op. 42, spr. 108–109v.

letters he wrote her between 1895 and his death in 1931.[98] Nevertheless, she was left to raise their four children alone, as Herman was almost always away, either in the Austrian parliament or, later, once Poland had independence after World War I, in the Polish Sejm (the lower house); and when he was not in parliament, he was representing his party or country abroad.[99] He stayed, however, genuinely engaged in his children lives, albeit mostly by mail. Herman died on February 26, 1931, the day he returned from a meeting of the executive of the International Socialist Bureau in Zurich. Hermina was the only one of the Lazarus children to survive World War II, living under an assumed identity in the countryside near Warsaw. She died in 1951 in Bytom, Poland.

After finishing their education at Niedziałkowska's gymnasium, both Eleonora and Fryderyka secretly prepared for the gymnasium diploma, which was not available at private schools for girls at the time. Although their parents encouraged their sons to pursue higher education, they did not believe their daughters required it. Eleonora's dream was to get a baccalauréat at the Sorbonne,[100] as some students could start their education without it and complete it as the first part of their studies. She wanted to study microbiology, a new branch of science. Her father gave her a choice: she could either have the family estate in Ostrów or he would pay for her studies. He hoped she would choose Ostrów; she chose the Sorbonne.

In 1899, two years after women were allowed to attend the Lviv University Philosophy Faculty, and a year before they were allowed to study medicine there,[101] Eleonora entered the Science Faculty of the University of Paris (the Sorbonne). Only eight years earlier, in late 1891, Marie Curie had begun studying at the Sorbonne; and in 1906, she had become the first woman professor there. After completing her degree (fig. 2.25), Eleonora took a course in microbiology in November 1906–March 1907 at the Pasteur Institute in Paris (fig. 2.26 and fig. 2.27). Having won an internship, she stayed there until 1909, working in Giovanni Malfitano's laboratory, in the department headed by Amédée Borrel.[102] In 1910, the results of her work were published in an article in the *Annales de l'Institut Pasteur: journal de microbiologie*.[103]

Eleonora was also interested in photography and was given her first camera by her mother for her twenty-first birthday in 1898.[104] In 1904, during her Paris years, she participated in the Second Annual Photographic Exhibition in Lviv, organized by the Lviv Photographic Society.[105] Unfortunately, none of her photographs from the exhibit have survived.

---

98 Herman Diamand, *Pamiętnik Hermana Diamanda zebrany z wyjątków listów do żony* (Kraków: Tow. Uniwersytetu Robotniczego [TUR], Oddział im. Adama Mickiewicza w Krakowie, 1932), accessed June 5, 2022, https://www.sbc.org.pl/dlibra/doccontent?id=14023.
99 Ibid.; see also: Ewa Herbst, "Herman Diamand—on the 90th Anniversary of His Death," *Kwartalnik Historii Żydów* 287, no. 3 (2023): 549–576.
100 French national academic qualification obtained after secondary education.
101 See chapter 1.
102 Scientific Information Resource Center (CeRIS), Library and Archives, Pasteur Institute, 2023.
103 Eleonora Lazarus, "Sur la Protéolyse de la bactéridie charbonneuse," *Annales de l'Institut Pasteur: journal de microbiologie / publiées sous le patronage de M. Pasteur par E. Duclaux*, no. 7 (1910): 577–594.
104 LNNBU, fond 44, op. 30 part 1, spr. 194v.
105 Iryna Kotlobulatova, *Yevreis'ki fotohrafy ta fotostudii L'vova (1860–1939)* (Lviv: Vydavnytstvo Staroho Leva, 2024), 245. On pages 244–248, there are several photographs by Eleonora Lazarus from Ewa Herbst's collection.

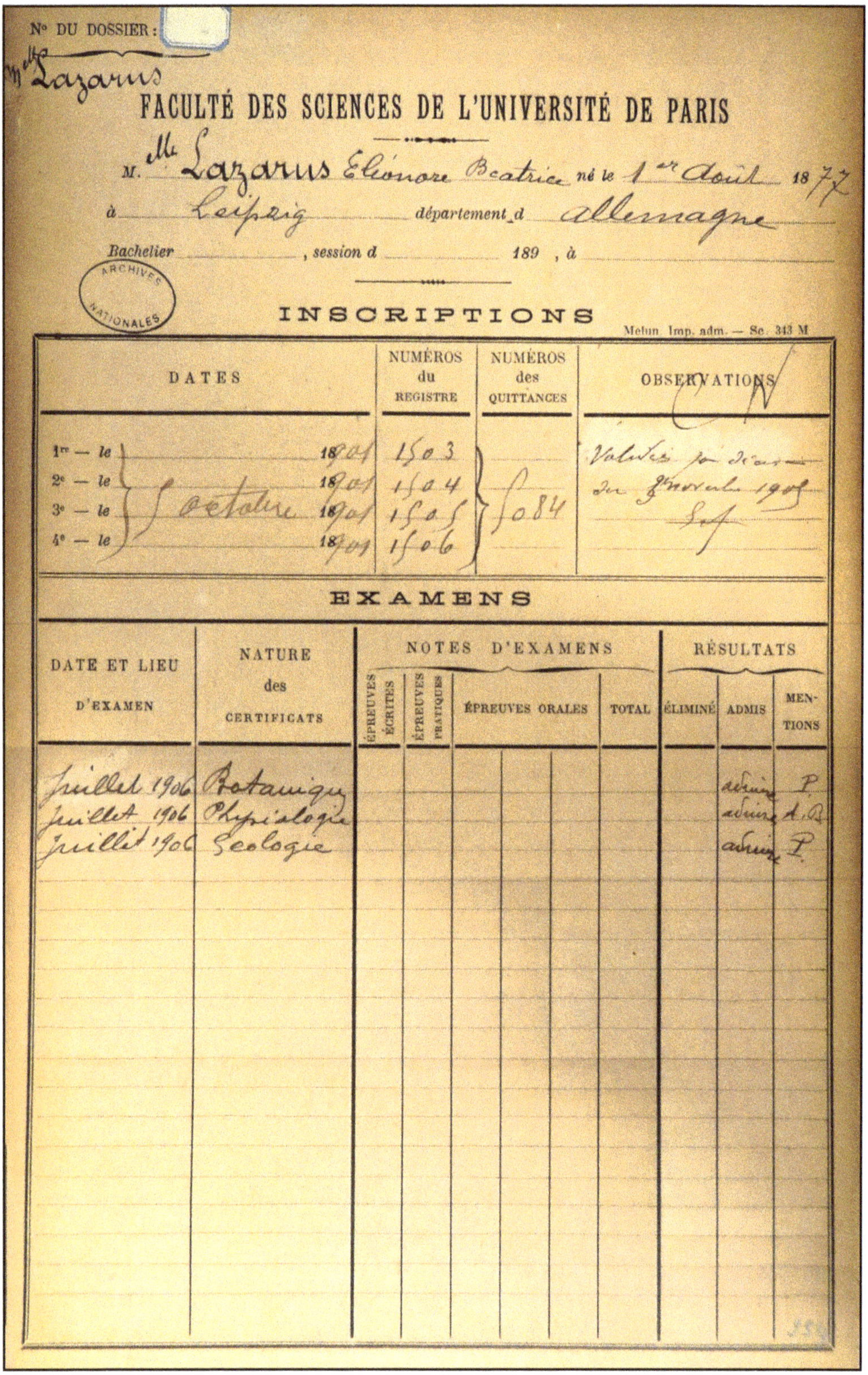

N° DU DOSSIER :

Mlle Lazarus

FACULTÉ DES SCIENCES DE L'UNIVERSITÉ DE PARIS

M. Mlle Lazarus Eléonore Beatrice né le 1er août 1877

à Leipzig département d Allemagne

Bachelier , session d 189 , à

ARCHIVES NATIONALES

INSCRIPTIONS

Melun. Imp. adm. — Sc. 343 M

DATES	NUMÉROS du REGISTRE	NUMÉROS des QUITTANCES	OBSERVATIONS
1re — le 5 octobre 1901	1503	5084	Validées par décision du 8 novembre 1905
2e — le 5 octobre 1901	1504		
3e — le 5 octobre 1901	1505		
4e — le 5 octobre 1901	1506		

EXAMENS

DATE ET LIEU D'EXAMEN	NATURE des CERTIFICATS	NOTES D'EXAMENS: ÉPREUVES ÉCRITES	ÉPREUVES PRATIQUES	ÉPREUVES ORALES	TOTAL	RÉSULTATS: ÉLIMINÉ	ADMIS	MENTIONS
Juillet 1906	Botanique						admis	P.
Juillet 1906	Physiologie						admis	A.B.
Juillet 1906	Géologie						admis	P.

Figure 2.25. Courses taken by Eleonora Lazarus at Sorbonne. Left - final exams, right – laboratories. Archives Nationales de France AJ/16/5707.

TRAVAUX PRATIQUES

TRIMESTRES	NATURE des TRAVAUX PRATIQUES	NUMÉROS des quittances.	SOMMES VERSÉES	TRIMESTRES	NATURE des TRAVAUX PRATIQUES	NUMÉROS des quittances.	SOMMES VERSÉES
	Année scolaire 1899-1900				*Année scolaire 1900-1901*		
	Immatriculé	6412	30		Immatriculé	7676	30
1ᵉʳ	Géologie	6412	10	1ᵉʳ	Botanique	7676	2f
	Botanique	6412	1f		Physiologie	7676	2f
	Zoologie	6412	2f		Géologie	7676	1a
	Géologie	31	10		Botanique	296	2f
2ᵉ	Botanique	31	1f	2ᵉ	Physiologie	296	2f
	Zoologie	31	2f		Géologie	296	10
	Géologie	1153	10		Botanique	1783	2f
3ᵉ	Botanique	1153	1f	3ᵉ	Physiologie	1783	2f
	Zoologie	1153	2f		Géologie	1781	10
	Géologie	2659	10		Botanique	2990	2f
4ᵉ	Botanique	2659	1f	4ᵉ	Physiologie	2990	2f
	Zoologie	2659	2f		Géologie	2990	10
	Année scolaire 1901-1902				*Année scolaire 18 -18 .*		
	Immatriculé	5891	30		Immatriculé		
1ᵉʳ	Botanique	5084	2f	1ᵉʳ			
	Physiologie	5891	2f				
	Embryologie	5891	2f				
	Botanique	5084	2f				
2ᵉ	Physiologie	671	2f	2ᵉ			
	Embryologie	671	2f				
	Physiologie	1799	2f				
3ᵉ	Embryologie	1799	2f	3ᵉ			
	Botanique	5084	2f				
4ᵉ	Botanique	5084	2f	4ᵉ			

However, a large number of her glass-plate negatives survived the war. One of her most interesting photographs is of the City Theater (Teatr Miejski, inaugurated in October 1900; presently, Lviv Opera; fig. 2.28) at night. The picture seems to be taken at an angle from the balcony or window of 39 Karl Ludwig Street (later Legionów; presently, Prospekt Svobody)—Maurycy's and Betti Diamand house, the parents of Herman Diamand, her brother-in-law, and Aleksander Diamand, her future husband. Eleonara also published a couple of children's books.

While living in Paris, she was active in the Foreign Union to Aid Political Victims,[106] established in 1905, and moved in Polish political émigré circles. The people she knew were insurgents from the 1863 January Uprising, communards (among them general Walery Wróblewski),[107] young socialists, and Polish independence activists. She hiked in the Alps with some of them.

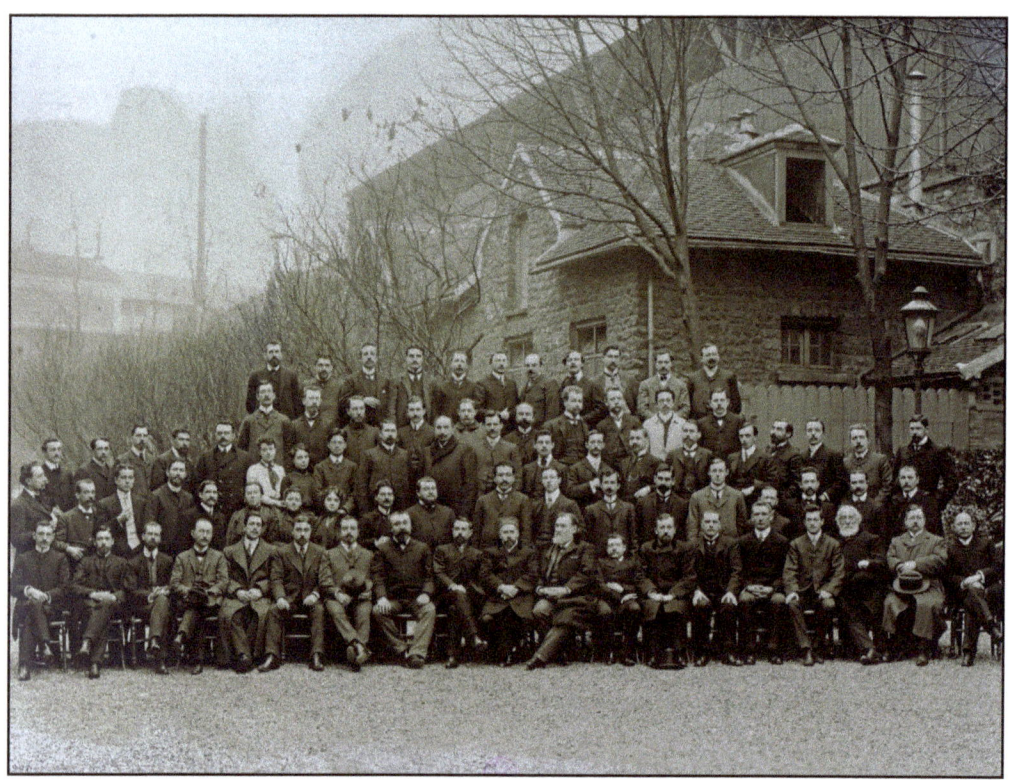

Figure 2.26. Microbiology course (*Grand Cours de microbiologie*), Pasteur Institute November 1906-March 1907. Photo: Institut Pasteur/Musée Pasteur.

---

106 Eleonora Lazarus, "Zagraniczny Związek Pomocy dla Ofiar Politycznych," *Kurjer lwowski*, August 3, 1907, 4–5.
107 Walery Wróblewski (1836–1908)—a commander during the January Uprising and a Paris Commune general.

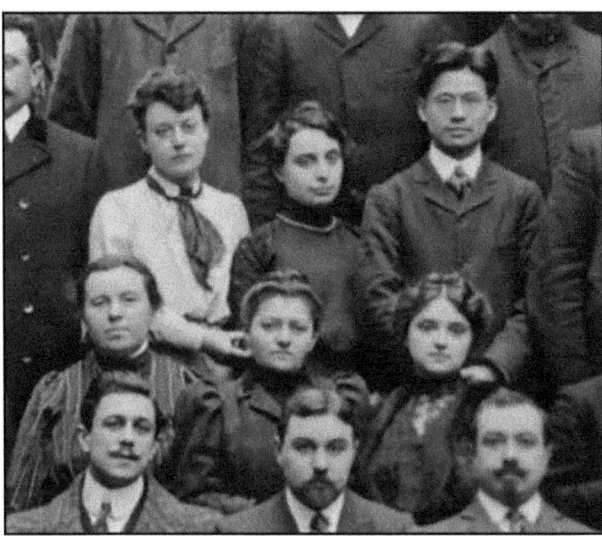

Figure 2.27. Enlargement of a portion of the photo 2.26. Eleonora Lazarus standing in the third row, in the middle.

After Walery Wróblewski's death in August 1908, Eleonora joined the committee organizing his funeral. Pretending to be his niece, she obtained a police permit for his funeral at the Père-Lachaise Cemetery in Paris, showing financial resources to pay for his grave.[108] Thousands of people took part in the funeral procession.

Living once again in Lviv, in 1909 Eleonora married Aleksander Diamand, the younger brother of Herman. Having given birth to three children between 1910 and 1914, and with the disruption of World War I, she never returned to her profession. However, she stayed active in causes close to her heart and worked on behalf of political prisoners. In 1911, she became the co-organizer and secretary of the Society for the Welfare of Political Prisoners, created on the initiative of Aleksandra Piłsudska,[109] the second wife of Józef Piłsudski.[110] According to Aleksandra Piłsudska, members of the society concealed very thin saws,

---

108 The following documents confirm family stories about Eleonora's role in organizing Walery Wróblewski's funeral: Jerzy W. Borejsza, *Patriota bez paszportu*, 3rd ed. (Warsaw: Neriton, 2008), 231; Leonard Dubacki, "Walery Wróblewski (1836–1908)," *Przegląd Socjalistyczny*, accessed June 16, 2023, http://przeglad-socjalistyczny.pl/wielcy-socjalici/189-aziemski; Andrzej Biernat, ed., *Inskrypcje grobów polskich na cmentarzach w Paryżu – Père Lachaise* (Warsaw: ZOiKZP-O, 1991), 73, according to which Eleonora purchased the cemetery plot on August 15, 1908 (D. C. = Dossier de la concession in the Office of the Conservator of Père-Lachaise Cemetary). I thank Dr. Marcin Starnawski for bringing to my attention Jerzy Borejsza's book and Barbara Bułat at the Jagiellonian Library in Kraków for an extensive search that confirmed Eleonora's purchase of the plot at the Père Lachaise cemetery.

109 Polish: Towarzystwo Opieki nad Więźniami Politycznymi; Aleksandra Piłsudska, *Wspomnienia* (Warsaw: Instytut Prasy i Wydawnictw "Novum," 1989), 124–125.

110 Józef Piłsudski (1867–1935)—Polish revolutionary and statesman. Early in his political career he became a leader of the Polish Socialist Party (PPS); he formed the Polish Legions, which fought on the side of Austria-Hungary against Russia during World War I; he was independent Poland's first chief of state (1918–1922); from 1920, he was the first marshal of Poland. He is considered father of the Second Polish Republic.

for cutting prison bars, in the parcels they sent to Polish political prisoners who had been deported to penal colonies in Siberia.[111]

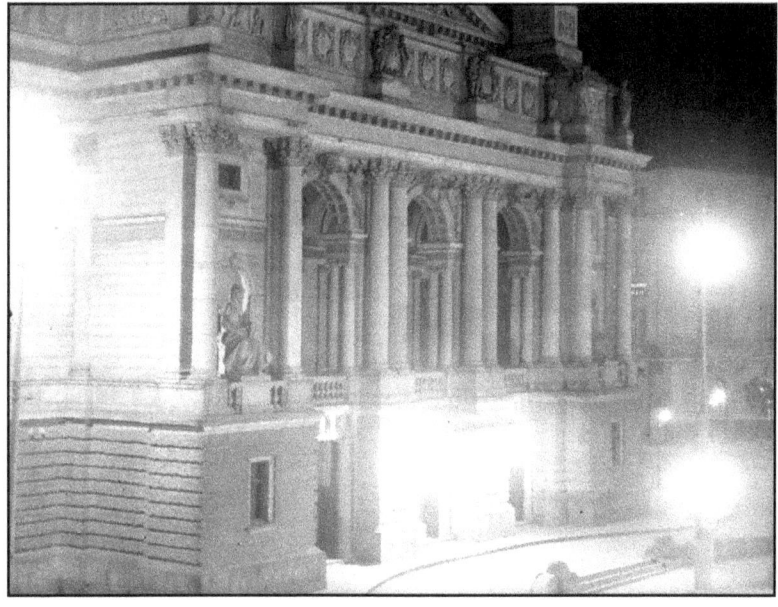

Figure 2.28. The City Theater (presently Lviv Opera). Photo: Eleonora Lazarus, circa 1900–1910. Author's collection.

Eleonora told her children that she hid false passports, money, and her address in the covers of the books she sent these men. As a result, a bearded and devastated escapee would sometimes show up at the door. The first thing he would do was gather up one of the children in his arms, perhaps yearning for his own. Eleonora was concerned about hygiene, but she would not deny the man his moment of happiness. Later, in the 1930s, Eleonora was the secretary of the League for Defense of Human and Civil Rights in Lviv.[112] She was also a member of the executive committee of the Jewish Hospital Council.

During the "Great Aktion" of August 1942, Eleonora and Aleksander Diamand were taken from their home in Lviv. He was most likely taken to the Janowska concentration camp and either killed there or transferred to the Belzec (Bełżec) extermination camp; there is no information about his fate. She was taken to the grounds of the Jewish Hospital, where women were held. Someone there recognized and saved her. She was given an injection, lost consciousness and was removed from the area with the dead. Later, she lived under an assumed identity in Warsaw. She was murdered around August 1, 1944, when German troops massacred the population of the Wola district in response to the start of the Warsaw Uprising.

---

111 Aleksandra Piłsudska, *Wspomnienia*, 125.
112 Polish: Liga Obrony Praw Człowieka i Obywatela.

Maurycy's and Róża's youngest daughter, Fryderyka,[113] influenced by the social and political currents prevailing at the time, wanted to become a teacher and prepared for it in secret, as her parents thought that neither a teacher-training college comprised of girls from various social backgrounds nor work itself were suitable for a young woman of her standing. When staying with Eleonora in Paris, she used her time there to study, and later she studied in Berlin at the Pestalozzi-Fröbel-Haus,[114] the first academic institution to offer women training as kindergarten teachers.[115]

Her career had to wait, however, as she needed to take care of her ailing mother; and after her mother's death in 1904, Fryderyka looked after her father for a while. From 1905, she worked with poor and orphaned children in Włochy (outside Warsaw), and later she co-organized community centers for children in Warsaw's working-class districts. After a while, she moved back to Galicia. However, she needed an internship to become a teacher there, which she was not able to get due to her being both Jewish and a member of the Social Democratic Party of Galicia. She eventually secured a position at the Baron de Hirsch Foundation's school in Tarnów. Shortly before World War I, she visited important educational institutions in Europe, including Montessori schools. During World War I, she was in charge of a Lviv orphanage and community center[116] for the orphans of soldiers of the Polish Legions (which fought on the side of Austria-Hungary in World War I), a military organization created in Galicia in August 1914.

After the war, in 1919–1920, Fryderyka worked in the newly opened Our Home (Nasz Dom)[117] in Pruszków, near Warsaw (fig. 2.29), established and headed by Maryna Falska and run according to the pedagogical methods of Janusz Korczak,[118] who himself spent one or two days a week there. It was a home for the children of workers who had fallen during World War I and children from poor families. Fryderyka was briefly in charge of a Home for Abandoned Jewish Children at 27 Ogrodowa Street in Warsaw, and she remained in Janusz Korczak's circle. After returning to Lviv, she studied to qualify as a high school biology teacher and worked in the Adam Mickiewicz Private Humanistic Gymnasium and later at elementary schools—her old dream. In parallel with her life as a teacher, Fryderyka was

---

113 Stanisław Konarski, "Lazarusówna Fryderyka," in *Polski Słownik Biograficzny*, ed. Franciszek Kubacz and Ignacy Piotr Legatowicz (Wroclaw-Warsaw-Kraków: Zakład Narodowy imienia Ossolińskich, Wydawnictwo Polskiej Akademii Nauk, 1971), 588–589.
114 Ibid.
115 "Big ideas since 1874," Pestalozzi-Fröbel-Haus, accessed June 7, 2023, https://www.pfh-berlin.de/en/article/big-ideas-1874.
116 Stanisław Konarski, "Lazarusówna Fryderyka,"
117 In fig. 2.29 "Józefa Dzięcioł, Maria Podwysocka, Maria Znamierowska i Fryderyka Lazarus w Naszym Domu w Pruszkowie," Museum of Warsaw, accessed December 22, 2022, https://kolekcje.muzeumwarszawy.pl/pl/obiekty/14725/. I thank Marta Ciesielska, Korczakianum's curator, for providing this information.
118 Maryna Falska (1877–1944) and Janusz Korczak (the pen name of Henryk Goldszmit [1878–1942]) were pedagogues; they each ran an orphanage according to Janusz Korczak's pedagogical methods. Maryna Falska died of a heart attack on September 7, 1944 when the Germans arrived to move the children. Janusz Korczak's orphanage was for Jewish children and was called the Children's Home (Dom Sierot). He was murdered in Treblinka in 1942 with his wards.

active in the Red Scouting's friendship circle[119] and sat on the board of the Workers' Society of Friends of Children.[120] She also wrote about twenty children's books.

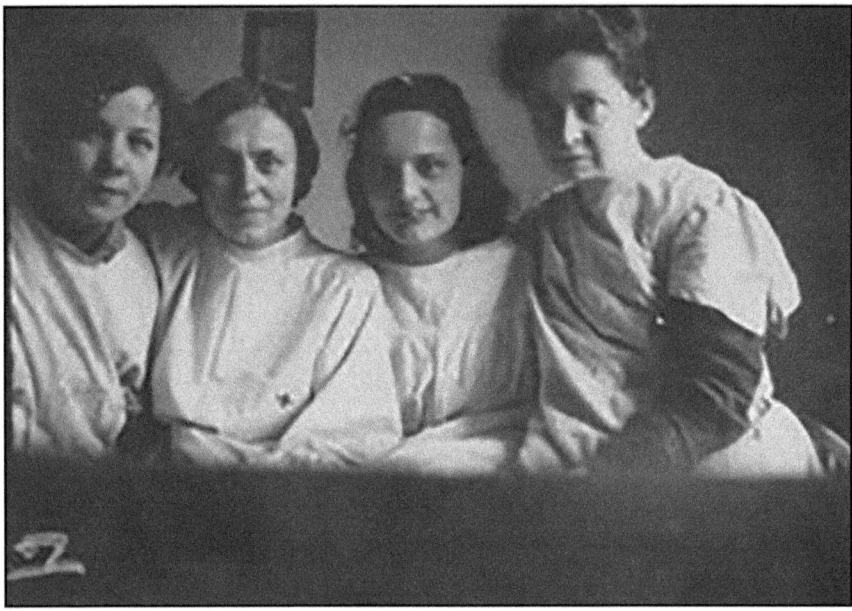

Figure 2.29. Fryderyka Lazarus first from right at Nasz Dom in 1919/1920. The others from the left are: Józefa Dzięcioł, Maria Podwysocka, and Maria Znamierowska. Korczakianum, Warsaw.

Fryderyka Lazarus was beloved by her students and, according to one of them, "legends circulated throughout the city about her nobility and her devotion to children" (fig. 2.30).[121] In August 1942, the time of the extermination of Lviv's Jews, she was taken from her home by the Germans. Realizing what was about to happen, as the district was already surrounded, she gathered the latest volumes of her books, ran to Janina Kelles-Krauz's[122] nearby house, and left them there. In the short letter she left, she wrote that at the worst moment of her life she was entrusting her with her life's work in the hope that it could still be useful for children. There is no information about how she died.

---

119 Polish: Koło Przyjaciół Czerwonego Harcerstwa.
120 Polish: Robotnicze Towarzystwo Przyjaciół Dzieci.
121 Miriam Lipa, "Fryderyka Lazarus ze Lwowa. Ratujmy wspomnienia," *Nowiny Kurier*, January 4, 1979, 4.
122 Janina Kelles-Krauz worked at the Ossolineum—a Polish cultural foundation, major archive, research center, and publishing house. Earlier in 1942, all of Herman Diamand's and his family's documents were deposited there.

4 stycznia 1979 — Nr 4 — Rok XXI (XXV)

Fryderyka Lazarus ze Lwowa

MIRIAM LIPA
(Holon)

Znana rodzina żydowskich magnatów i społeczników Maurycego LAZARUSA wiele dała państwu polskiemu, nie zatracając jednocześnie nigdy więzów z narodem żydowskim. Przy ul. Rapaporta we Lwowie został wybudowany przez tę rodzinę szpital żydowski i obok żydowski dom starców.

Fryderyka LAZARUS była nieodrodną córką swego szlachetnego ojca, Maurycego. Z przekonań socjalistka, członkini PPS-Lewicy. Po pierwszej wojnie światowej oddała swój posag Skarbowi wyzwolonej Polski. W owym czasie była wielką entuzjastką Piłsudskiego. Potem uważała go za zdrajcę głoszonych przez niego ideałów.

Uczyła w państwowej szkole dla żydowskiej młodzieży im. Króla Jana Sobieskiego, oraz w gimnazjach im. im. Olgi Filipi i Strzałkowskiej.

W całym mieście krążyły legendy o Jej szlachetności i wielkim oddaniu dzieciom. Gdy i do mnie doszła opinia o Niej,

miałam 11 lat i chodziłam do innej szkoły, w innej dzielnicy miasta i byłam o klasę wyżej, niż ta, w której Ona uczyła. Przestałam odrabiać lekcje bo chciałam się zrównać z Jej klasą i pod pozorem wstydu powtarzania roku w tej samej szkole, w następnym roku zostałam jej wychowanicą.

Gorąco wszystkie kochałyśmy Ją. Był to okres masowego zwalniania Żydów z państwowych stanowisk. I Jej groziło

RATUJMY WSPOMNIENIA

zwolnienie, szczególnie z powodu nie ukrywanego antagonizmu wobec Piłsudskiego. Dzięki temu, że prosiła by pozostawiono Ją bez uposażenia, aż do doprowadzenia swych podopiecznych do ukończenia podstawowej szkoły, pozostała na placówce, choć była szykanowana przez władze. Niewspółmierne i niespodziewane (kilka razy w tygodniu) naloty wizytacji nie potrafiły jednak znaleźć w jej pracy usterek. Dzieci naszej klasy miały wyjątkowy poziom przez Nią rozwijanej w nas, inteligencji. Jej działalność nie kończyła się na nauczaniu i służeniu nam przykładem. Była w kontakcie z różnymi zagranicznymi organizacjami społecznymi i stamtąd otrzymywała odzież dziecięcą, którą rozdzielała między ubogie dziewczynki naszej szkoły, znajdującej się w robotniczej dzielnicy miasta. W efekcie nie było wśród nas źle ubranych, lub chodzących w podartych butach, co było wówczas zjawiskiem powszechnym w innych szkołach.

Pisała książki dla dzieci. Wydawała je tzw. „Błękitna i Różowa Biblioteczka". Pod Jej

kierunkiem dzieci naszej klasy wydały również książkę, nakładem tegoż wydawnictwa, pod tytułem „Siódmoklasistki żeńskiej szkoły im. Króla Jana Sobieskiego we Lwowie". Każdy rozdział pisała inna dziewczynka. Były to wspomnienia z naszego życia szkolnego.

Po ukończeniu naszej nauki w szkole podstawowej, przez całe wakacje przygotowywała nas bezpłatnie do egzaminu wstępnego i 45 dziewczynek (na 48) z naszej klasy przy Jej wielkiej pomocy rozpoczęło naukę w gimnazjum „Kammerling". Dla niezamożnych dzieci wystarała się o zniżkę czesnego, innym wystarała się o korepetycje i w ten sposób pokrywały opłatę za naukę. Jeszcze wiele lat później chodziła na „wywiadówki" i razem z naszymi matkami cieszyła się lub smuciła usłyszaną opinią.

Kochałam ją tak prawie, jak Matkę. Marzyłam, że gdy będę miała w przyszłości męża i dzieci, postawię w salonie 2 fotele: jeden dla mojej Mamusi i drugi dla Niej.

Niestety nie ziściły się te plany. Hitler zabrał „oba fotele".

Często myślałam, jak uczcić pamięć tej świetlanej postaci. Dziś, jeśli Redakcja uzna powyższy list za materiał nadający się do umieszczenia na łamach prasowych, będę miała lżejsze sumienie, w nadziei, że jeszcze ktoś z małej garstki lwowian, pozostałych przy życiu po strasznej rzezi, również odda hołd Jej pamięci.

Choć żadnemu z nas nie brakuje wspomnień po naszych zamęczonych Najbliższych nie powinniśmy zapomnieć TAKICH POSTACI, jak FRYDERYKA LAZARUS.

Figure 2.30. Article about Fryderyka Lazarus by Miriam Lipa, one of her pupils. "Fryderyka Lazarus ze Lwowa," Nowiny Kurier, Israel, January 4, 1979.

Hugo

Little is known about Hugo Lazarus (1875–1916), the youngest son of Maurycy and Róża (fig. 2.31). He was a medical doctor who studied in Vienna and graduated in 1906 and later took some medical courses as a special student at the Lviv University.[123] During World War I, he served in the Austrian military hospitals and volunteered to take care of typhus patients during the epidemic. He lost his life to the disease in 1916.

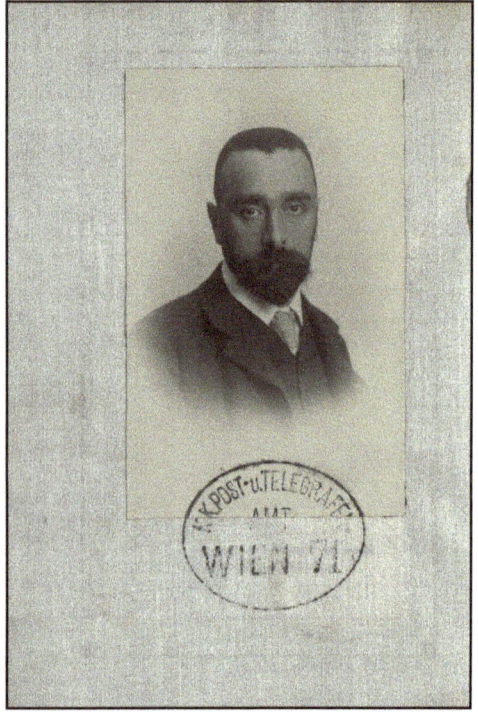 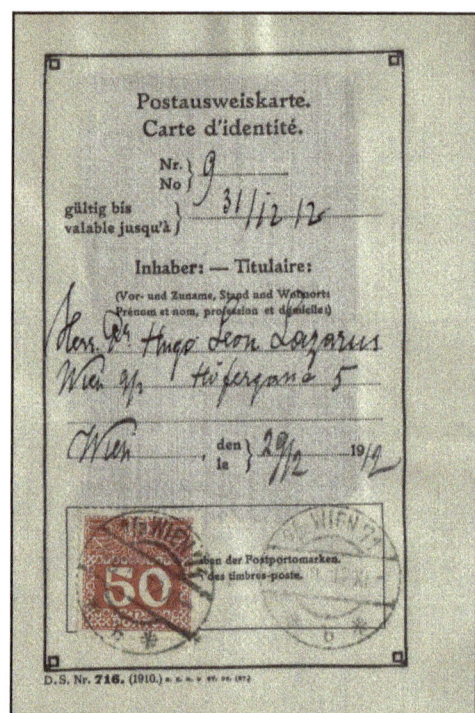

Figure 2.31. Identity card of Hugo Lazarus. Ossolineum, digital collection. Original in LNNBU, fond 44, op. 42, spr. 137.

***

Maurycy Lazarus lived to be eighty and died on April 30, 1912. His life spanned a period of great historical changes in Galicia, and in Europe as a whole. Those changes were even more pronounced for the Galician Jews.

Maurycy Lazarus grew up during the second half of the Jewish Enlightenment in a merchant family with the resources to send him to study in Vienna. He took an active part in the Spring of Nations and held to its ideals throughout his life. At first strongly attracted to Viennese liberal ideas, and counting on the fact that Jews were better

---

123 DALO, fond 26, op. 15 spr. 835.

protected there, he gradually came to see that the fate of Galician Jews was intimately connected with the fate of Poland. After the 1867 Constitution gave Jews equal rights, he increasingly engaged in political and social matters; and over the years, he became one of Lviv's most prominent citizens. An enormously talented businessman, he shared his wealth through acts of great generosity. The Jewish Hospital he envisioned was the most modern hospital in Galicia when it was founded, and it is still operating as a municipal hospital over 120 years later.

The path of each of Maurycy's children was very different from his own; and it was not always easy for him to accept their decisions, especially when it came to his daughters. There were conflicts and compromises, but the family was close, and when apart they constantly wrote to one another. Regardless of their various political views, each member of the family was committed to serving the community. The distance from the Vienna-inspired Jewish Enlightenment at the beginning of Maurycy Lazarus's adulthood to the radical ideas of the turn of the twentieth century that his children embraced may seem long, but it was traveled in this one remarkable man's lifetime.

Archival Sources

AGAD
Fond 300, sign. 516, case 504.

APP
Sign. 56/1924/0/-/19.

DALO
Fond 26, op. 15 spr. 835.

IKG
Matriken der Israelitischen Kultusgemeinde, 1784–1911.

HDA
Fond 252 (RUR IURP ŽO), kut. 14, br. 29701.

LNNBU
Fond 44, op. 30 part 1, spr. 194v
Fond 44, op. 42, spr. 108–109v.
Fond 44, op. 54, spr. 92.

TsDIAL
Fond 701, op. 1, spr. 113, f. 31, k. 25; fond 701, op. 1, spr. 118, f. 48, k. 642.
Fond 701, op. 4 od. Zb. 279.

WSTLA
WSTLA_LG_Zivilrechtssachen_A26_48T_24T_Todeserklärungen_48T_81_1957.

Bibliography

Bałaban, Majer. *Dzieje Żydów w Galicyi i w Rzeczypospolitej Krakowskiej 1772–1868*. Lwów: Księgarnia Polska B. Połonieckiego, 1914.

———. *Historia lwowskiej synagogi postępowej*. Lwów: Zarząd Synagogi Postępowej we Lwowie, 1937.

Biernat, Andrzej, ed. *Inskrypcje grobów polskich na cmentarzach w Paryżu – Père Lachaise*. Warsaw: ZOiKZP-O, 1991.

"Big Ideas since 1874." Pestalozzi-Fröbel-Haus. Accessed June 7, 2023. https://www.pfh-berlin.de/en/article/big-ideas-1874.

Borejsza, Jerzy W. *Patriota bez paszportu*. 3rd ed. Warsaw: Neriton, 2008.

Diamand, Herman. *Pamiętnik Hermana Diamanda zebrany z wyjątków listów do żony*. Kraków: Tow. Uniwersytetu Robotniczego (TUR), Oddział im. Adama Mickiewicza w Krakowie, 1932. Accessed June 5, 2022. https://www.sbc.org.pl/dlibra/doccontent?id=14023.

Dubacki, Leonard. "Walery Wróblewski (1836–1908)." Przegląd socjalistyczny. Accessed June 16, 2023. http://przeglad-socjalistyczny.pl/wielcy-socjalici/189-aziemski.

"Etyka miljonerów." *Kurjer lwowski*, March 5, 1901.

Feuerstein, Henryk. "Lazarus: życie i czyny żydowskiego filantropa." In *Almanach Żydowski wydany przez Hermana Stachla zawierający szereg artykułów wybitnych literatów, polityków i publicystów oraz życiorysy czołowych postaci Małopolski Wschodniej*, 216–219. Lwów: Wydawnictwo Kultura i Sztuka, 1937.

Gajak-Toczek, Małgorzata. "Męskie gimnazja państwowe we Lwowie w latach 1772–1914." *Acta Universitatis Lodziensis. Folia Litteraria Polonica* 13 (2010): 349–358.

Galicia 1891 Business Directory. JewishGen. Accessed August 14, 2023. https://www.jewishgen.org/databases/poland/galicia1891.htm.

Gelber, N. M. ed. *The Encyclopedia of the Jewish Diaspora, Poland Series: Lwów Volume (Lviv, Ukraine)*. Translated by Myra Yael Ecker. Jewish Gen. Last modified April 24, 2023. https://www.jewishgen.org/Yizkor/lviv/lviv.html.

Gotthard Deutsch and A. Kaminka. "Israelitische Allianz zu Wien." Jewish Encyclopedia. Accessed April 15, 2023. https://jewishencyclopedia.com/articles/8306-israelitische-allianz-zu-wien.

Grayson, Joshua. "Family Evidence Books: Another Treasure Trove." *Galitzianer* 25, no. 2 (2018): 8–11.

"The General Regional Exhibition of Galicia." Center for Urban History, Lviv. Accessed July 23, 2023. https://lia.lvivcenter.org/en/storymaps/exhibition-after/.

Herbst, Ewa. "Herman Diamand—on the 90th Anniversary of His Death." *Kwartalnik Historii Żydów* 287, no. 3 (2023): 125–152.

Ilustrowany Przewodnik po Lwowie i Powszechnej Wystawie Krajowej. Lwów: Towarzystwo dla Rozwoju i Upiększania Miasta, 1894.

Jakimyszyn-Gadocha, Anna. *W trosce o zdrowie żydowskiej społeczności Lwowa (1918–1939)*. Kraków: Wydawnictwo Austeria, 2021.

"Józefa Dzięcioł, Maria Podwysocka, Maria Znamierowska i Fryderyka Lazarus w Naszym Domu w Pruszkowie." Museum of Warsaw. Accessed December 22, 2022. https://kolekcje.muzeumwarszawy.pl/pl/obiekty/14725/.

Kaliński, Janusz. "Bankowość austriacka na ziemiach polskich." In *Między stabilizacją a ekspansją. System Finansowy w służbie modernizacji*, edited by J. Łazor, and W. Morawski, 269–284. N.p.: Gajt Wydawnictwo S. C., 2014.

Konarski, Stanisław. "Lazarusówna Fryderyka." In *Polski Słownik Biograficzny*, edited by Franciszek Kubacz and Ignacy Piotr Legatowicz, 588–589. Wroclaw-Warsaw-Kraków: Zakład Narodowy imienia Ossolińskich, Wydawnictwo Polskiej Akademii Nauk, 1971.

Kotlobulatova, Iryna. *Yevreis'ki fotohrafy ta fotostudii L'vova (1860–1939)*. Lviv: Vydavnytstvo Staroho Leva, 2023.

Księga adresowa Król. Stoł. Miasta Lwowa 1894. sbc.org. Accessed August 14, 2023. https://www.sbc.org.pl/dlibra/applet/Content/9432?handler=djvu_html5&file=%2FContent%2F9432%2Fimg_0088.djvu.

Księga adresowa Król. Stoł. Miasta Lwowa 1897. sbc.org. Accessed August 14, 2023. https://www.mtg-malopolska.org.pl/images/skany/ksiega_adresowa_1897/ksiega_adresowa_1897.pdf.

Księga Adresowa Król. Stoł. Miasta Lwowa 1902. Lwów: Wydawca Fr. Reichman, 1902.

Księga Pamiątkowa Towarzystwa "Bratniej Pomocy" Słuchaczów Politechniki we Lwowie. Lwów: Towarzystwo "Bratniej Pomocy" Słuchaczów Politechniki, 1897.

Kudła, Lucyna. "Gimnazjaliści galicyjskiej doby autonomicznej. Charakterystyka społeczności." *Annales Academiae Paedagogicae Cracoviensis* 4 (2005): 97–113.

Lazarus, Eleonora. "Sur la Protéolyse de la bactéridie charbonneuse." *Annales de l'Institut Pasteur: journal de microbiologie* / publiées sous le patronage de M. Pasteur par E. Duclaux, no. 7 (1910): 577–594.

Lazarus, Eleonora. "Zagraniczny Związek Pomocy dla Ofiar Politycznych." *Kurjer lwowski*, August 3, 1907.

Lazarus, Moritz. *Juden als Ackerbauern: ein Beitrag zur Lösung der sozialen Frage der Juden in Galizien*. Lemberg: n.p., 1885.

Lehman, Matthias B. *The Baron: Maurice de Hirsch and the Jewish nineteenth century*. Stanford: Stanford University Press, 2022.

"Lemberg." *Die Wahrheit*, May 3, 1912.

Lipa, Miriam. "Fryderyka Lazarus ze Lwowa. Ratujmy wspomnienia." *Nowiny Kurier*, January 4, 1979.

Łapot, Mirosław. "Rozwój żydowskiego szkolnictwa świeckiego we Lwowie w latach 1772–1879." *Prace Naukowe Akademii im. Jana Długosza w Częstochowie. Pedagogika* 22 (2013): 383–398.

Manekin, Rachel. "Politics, Religion and National Identity: The Galician Jewish Vote in the 1873 Parliamentary Elections." In *Focusing on Galicia: Jews, Poles and Ukrainians 1772–1918*. Polin Studies in Polish Jewry, vol. 12, edited by Israel Bartal and Antony Polonsky, 100–119. Oxford: The Littman Library of Jewish Civilization, 1999.

———. "Shomer Yisra'el." YIVO Encyclopedia of Jews in Eastern Europe. Accessed March 22, 2023. https://yivoencyclopedia.org/article.aspx/Shomer_Yisrael.

Mehrer, Henryk. *Szpital lwowskiej gminy wyznaniowej izraelickiej fundacyi Maurycego Lazarusa*. Lwów: Szpital Lwowskiej Gminy Wyzn. Izraelickiej, 1906.

Meus, Konrad. *Izba Handlowa i Przemysłowa we Lwowie (1850–1918) Instytucja i ludzie*. Kraków: Wydawnictwo Naukowe Instytutu Pedagogicznego, 2021.

Morawski, Wojciech. "Akcyjny Bank Hipoteczny SA we Lwowie." In *Słownik Historyczny Bankowości Polskiej do 1939 roku*, 89–90. Warsaw: Muza SA, 1998.

Neue Freie Presse, no 5051, September 19, 1878, 16.

"Nowa bożnica." *Kurjer lwowski*, April 1, 1908.

"Nowy szpital żydowski we Lwowie." *Kurjer lwowski*, June 8, 1903.

"The Pavilions of the Galician General Regional Exhibition of 1894." Forgotten Galicia. Accessed July 13, 2019. https://forgottengalicia.com/the-pavilions-of-the-galician-general-regional-exhibition-of-1894/.

Piłsudska, Aleksandra. *Wspomnienia*. Warsaw: Instytut Prasy i Wydawnictw "Novum," 1989.

Rosco-Bogdanowicz, Marian. *Wspomnienia*. Kraków: Wydawnictwo Literackie, 1959.

"Schloß Odrau, 700 Jahre Herrschaftssitz." Alte Heimat. Last modified September 15, 2009. https://www.kuhlaendchen.de/media/bilder/hk-odrau/SchlossOdrau.pdf.

Sroka, Łukasz T. *In the Light of Vienna: Jews in Lviv—Between Tradition and Modernisation (1867–1914)*. Berlin: Peter Lang, 2018.

———. *Rada Miejska we Lwowie w okresie autonomii galicyjskiej. Studium o elicie władzy*. Kraków: Wydawnictwo Naukowe Uniwersytetu Pedagogicznego, 2012.

———. "Members of the 'Leopolis' Humanitarian Society in Lvov (1899–1938): A Group Portrait." *Scripta Judaica Cracoviensia* 12 (2014): 99–119.

Statuta c.k. uprzyw. galicyjskiego akcyjnego Banku hipotecznego. Lwów: Drukiem Kornela Pillera, 1867.

Śliż, Małgorzata. *Galicyjscy Żydzi na drodze do równouprawnienia 1848–1914: aspekt prawny procesu emancypacji żydów w Galicji*. Kraków: Księgarnia Akademicka, 2006.

"Siedemdziesiąte urodziny." *Kurjer lwowski*, October 25, 1902.

Spitzer, Solomon. *Maurycy Baron Hirsch i jego działalność filantropijna*. Kraków: Drukiem Józefa Fischera, 1891.

Szematyzm królestwa Galicyi i Lodomeryi z wielkiem księstwem krakowskiem na rok 1872. Lwów: z drukarni E. Winiarza, 1872.

Szematyzm Królestwa Galicyi i Lodomeryi z Wielkiem Ksiestwem Krakowskiem na rok 1881. Lwów: Nakładem Galic. C. K. Namiestnictwa, 1881.

Szematyzm Królestwa Galicyi i Lodomeryi z Wielkim Księstwem Krakowskiem na rok 1892. Lwów: Nakładem C. K. Namiestnictwa, 1892.

Szematyzm Królestwa Galicyi i Lodomeryi z Wielkim Księstwem Krakowskiem na rok 1912. Lwów: Nakładem Prezydyum C. K. Namiestnictwa, 1912.

"Szomer Israel we Lwowie." Muzeum Historii Żydów Polskich POLIN. Accessed April 29, 2023. https://sztetl.org.pl/pl/miejscowosci/l/703-lwow/101-organizacje-i-instytucje-spoleczne/81036-szomer-israel-we-lwowie.

"Telegramy 'Kurjera lwowskiego'. Wiedeń 12 Marca." *Kurjer lwowski*, March 13, 1898.

"Z działalnosci wiedeńskiej 'Allianz' dla Galicyi." *Jedność*, May 20, 1910.

Zalewski, Andrew. "Soaring Hopes of 1848. Demonstrations and Petitions." *Galitzianer* 27, no. 2 (2020): 9–16.

———. "Jewish Petitioners. The Plan to Divide Galicia." *Galitzianer* 27, no. 4 (2020): 21–24.

———. "Jewish Marriages Revisited." *Galitzianer* 28, no. 2 (2021): 9–15.

Chapter 3

The Jewish Hospital in Lemberg/Lwów/Lviv: Its Architecture and Architects

Sergey R. Kravtsov

The Jewish Hospital, which today houses the municipal maternity hospital, is a distinctive and important landmark (fig. 3.1). The building was planned, designed, built, and equipped at the behest of the Maurycy Lazarus Foundation. Its construction in 1898–1903 marked a high point in providing the Jewish community with a state-of-the-art facility. The hospital's design is a celebration of the founders' identity, the Jewish community, and the professional thought and labor which has made this building inseparable from Lviv's urban fabric. Many citizens take the hospital for granted: it is simply part of the city, the place where they or their children were born or healed. However, the hospital's story is complex and vital for an understanding of how and why people make their work matter and go on.

The History of Jewish Hospitals in Lviv

The city of Lviv was founded in 1250–1256 by King Daniel of Galicia and Volhynia (1201–1264), who reigned from 1253 to 1264. It was named for his son Leo (Lev, ca. 1228–ca. 1301). The High Castle was built first, and a suburb grew at the foot of the Castle Mount. There is no evidence of a Jewish settlement that early in Lviv. However, the Jewish settlement in the vicinity is believed to be as old as that of the Ruthenians (Ukrainians) and the Armenians—which dates back almost to the very beginnings of the city—and whose early affinity to the place is proved by the antiquity of their churches.[1]

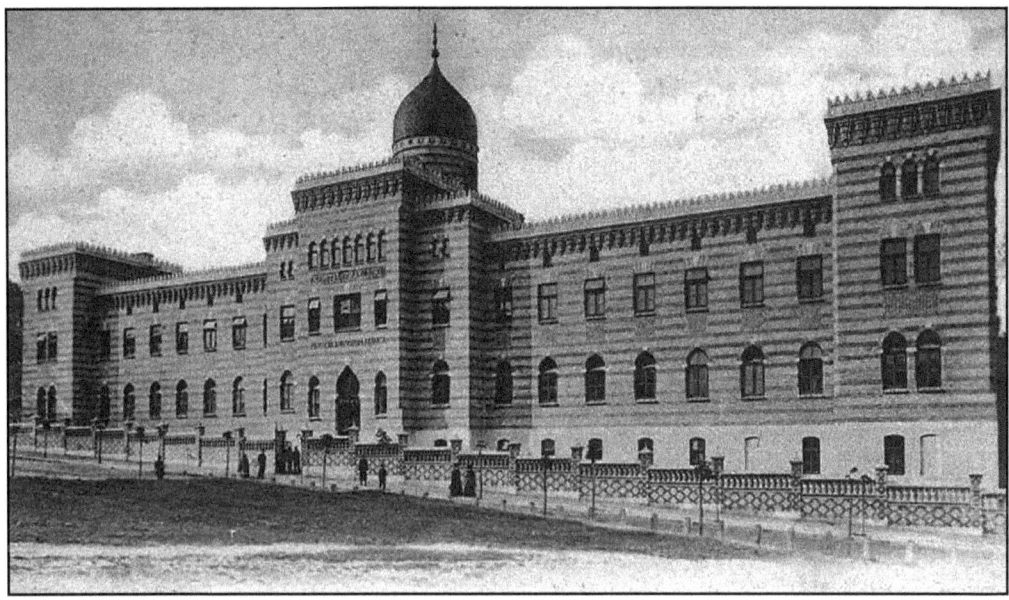

Figure 3.1. The Jewish Hospital, view from southeast. Photo Marek Münz, 1904. Henryk Mehrer, *Szpital lwowskiej gminy wyznaniowej izraelickiej fundacyi Maurycego Lazarusa* (Lwów: Szpital Lwowskiej Gminy Wyzn. Izraelickiej, 1906), 7.

Jews were first mentioned in Lviv in 1356, after the division of Galicia-Volhynia between the Kingdom of Poland and the Grand Duchy of Lithuania, and when, with the Magdeburg Law, the Polish king Casimir III, known as Casimir the Great (r. 1333–1370), granted the city autonomy. Under this law, Roman Catholics had full rights, while Jews were considered one of the city's "nations." These included Armenians, Saracens, Tatars, Ruthenians, and unspecified others, all of whom had the right to trial according to their own laws, under the supervision of the city judge.[2] Most scholars recognize that Casimir the Great's charter referred to the new city which was founded, planned, and subsequently surrounded by a wall to the south of the old one. This new city received the name of its predecessor, which was then demoted to the status of an unfortified suburb. Medieval Lviv became an important node of a far-reaching trade network, a crossroads between Crimea, Hungary, Lithuania, Moldavia, Muscovy, Turkey, Persia, and Western and Northern Europe.[3]

---

1 This view was first presented by Józef Bartołomiej Zimorowicz in his *Leopolis triplex* (1665–1672). Cf. Bartołomiej Zimorowicz, *Potriynyi L'viv: Leopolis Triplex*, Ukrainian trans. Natalia Tsariova (Lviv: Tsentr Yevropy, 2002), 50–51.
2 Miron Kapral, ed., *Privilegia Civitatis Leopoliensis (XIV–XVIII Saec.)* (Lviv: Dokumental'na skarbnytsia L'vova, 1998), 27–28.
3 Eleonora Nadel-Golobič, "Armenians and Jews in Medieval Lvov: Their Role in Oriental Trade, 1400–1600," *Cahiers du Monde Russe et Soviétique* 20, nos. 3–4 (1979): 354–59.

The Jewish Quarter occupied the southeastern corner of the walled city of Lviv. In 1367, its Jews received from King Casimir the Great a special privilege, which granted them internal autonomy, freedom of worship, and state protection against persecution. They formed a separate community—referred to as the "Communitas Judaeorum intra moenia habitantum" (Community of Jews living within the walls) in the city records. The suburban community was independent from its downtown sister, having its own elders, rabbis, synagogues, ritual baths, and guilds, while sharing the same cemetery from at least 1414. For centuries, there was rivalry between the two communities, and it was only in the eighteenth century that they united, each electing an equal number of council members and integrating all offices and finances.[4]

Lviv, as a part of Galicia, was annexed by the Habsburg Monarchy in 1772. Emperor Joseph II (1741–1790), who reigned from 1780 to 1790, abolished the Magdeburg Law in 1787, and the Lviv municipality was subordinated to the Galician governorate. The city walls were dismantled, its moats filled in, and the historical suburbs, now administered as districts, merged with the city's medieval nuclei into a larger urban entity.[5]

The first Jewish hospital, which probably served also as a hospice and shelter for travelers, was founded in about 1600 by a community elder, Mordechai son of Yitzhak, in the Jewish quarter within the city walls. Located on plot 254,[6] south of the Old Synagogue and west of the city's arsenal, that hospital was razed in 1795 because of its poor condition. In the early nineteenth century, the subsequent Jewish hospital was built beyond the city walls on a plot adjoining the Jewish cemetery (fig. 3.2). The hospital was financed from private donations and by a charity established by Isaac Waringer (1741–1817). In 1804, it had four rooms and thirty-six beds. In 1847, it acquired a maternity wing, bequeathed by the Orthodox rabbi Jacob Meshulam Ornstein (1775–1839) and his wife Sarah. With two more houses facing present Bazarna and Rappaport Streets, the hospital grew to twenty-eight rooms by 1902. Sixteen of these rooms served as outpatient clinics, offices, and physicians' apartments, while the other twelve housed eighty-two beds. It was a humble facility where patients could observe funeral processions from the windows. A shabby morgue, built in 1806, included the guard's family apartment, and his children played outside. The historian Majer Bałaban (1877–1942) also mentions scores of rats occasionally damaging corpses prepared for funerals.[7]

---

4 Majer Bałaban, *Dzielnica żydowska: jej dzieje i zabytki* (Lwów: Towarzystwo miłośników przeszłości Lwowa, 1909), 16–19.
5 Markian Prokopovych, *Habsburg Lemberg: Architecture, Public Space, and Politics in the Galician Capital, 1772–1914* (West Lafayette: Purdue University Press, 2009), 19–31.
6 Plot numberings gave way to street addresses in the nineteenth century.
7 Majer Bałaban, "Szpital żydowski we Lwowie," *Wschód* 108 (1902): 4.

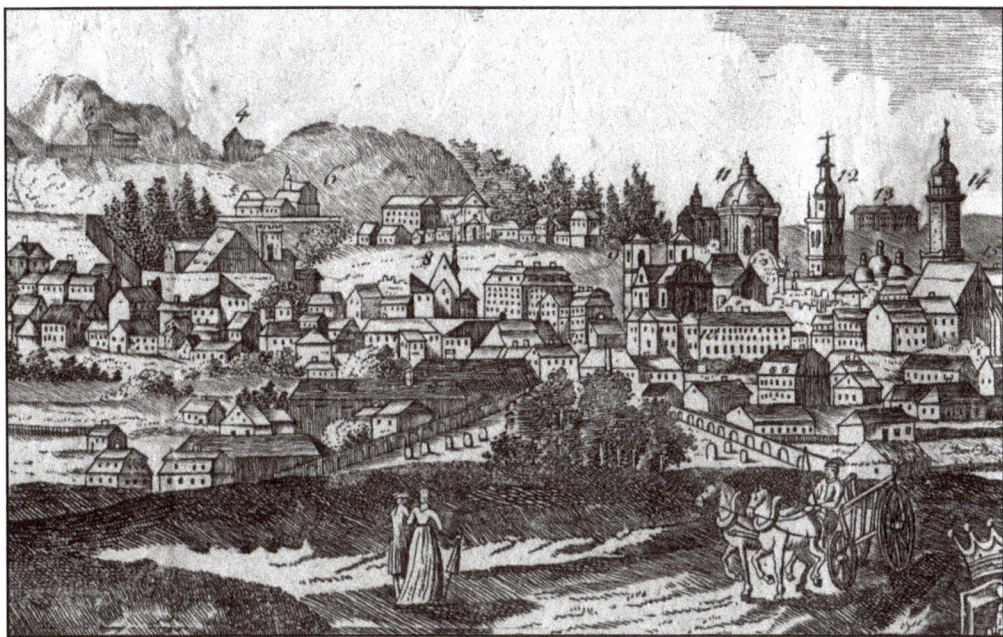

Figure 3.2. View of Lviv from west, fragment. From the guild book of soap makers, 1807. The Jewish hospital building is probably to the right (south) of the cemetery wall. Digital Archives in Opava, collection: Cech mydlářů Olomouc, M 3–21, no. 10.

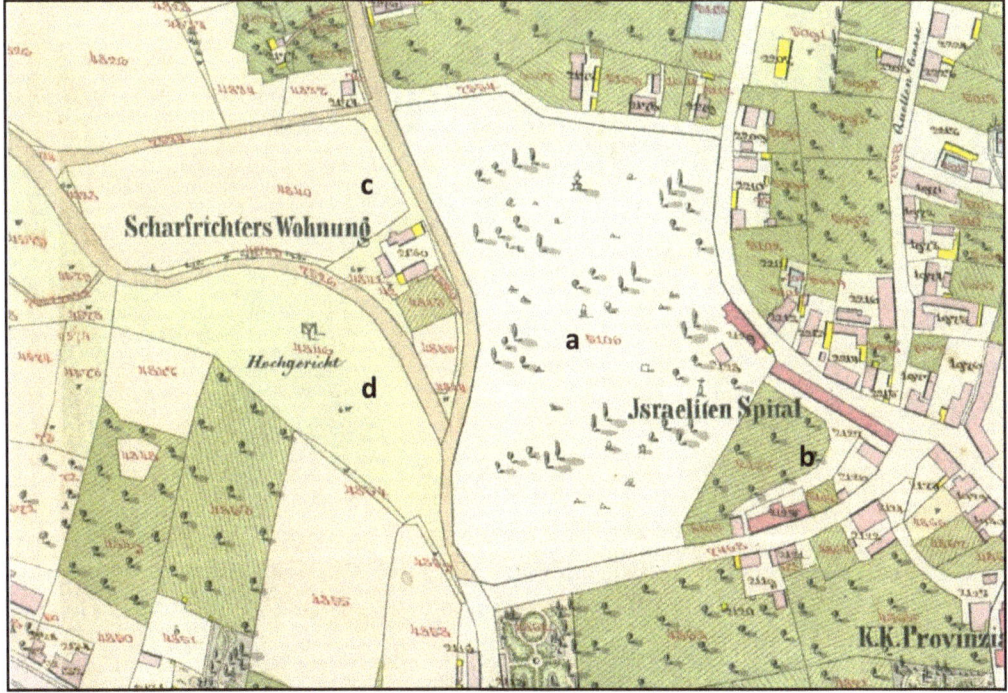

Figure 3.3. The Jewish Hospital and vicinity. Cadastral map from 1849/1853, fragment. a. Old Jewish Cemetery; b. Jewish Hospital; c. Hangman's quarters; d. Execution Mount. TsDIAL, fond 186, op. 8, spr. 628a.

94 | Sergey R. Kravtsov

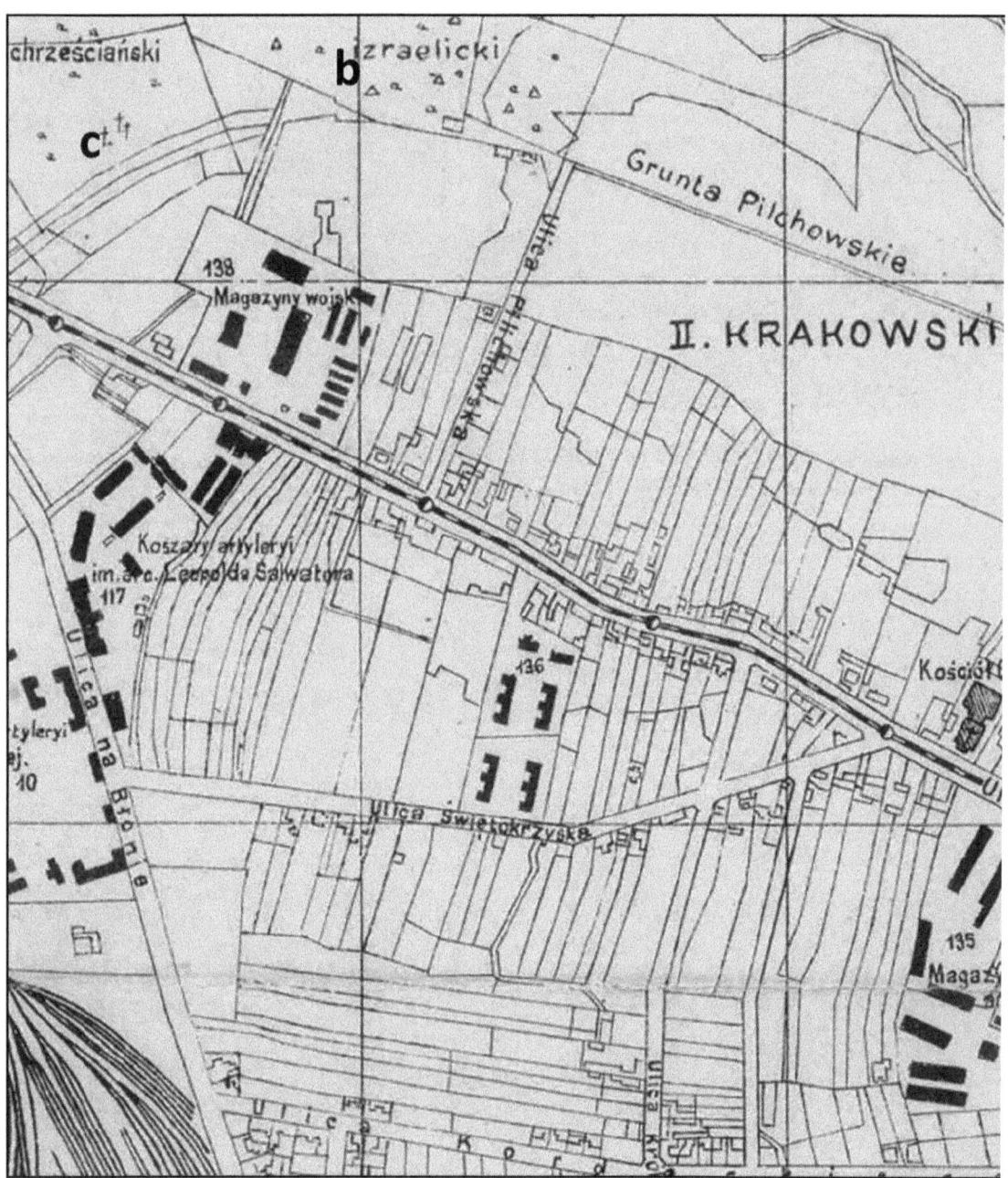

Figure 3.4. The Jewish Hospital and vicinity. City plan, 1910, fragment. a. Old Jewish Cemetery; b. New Jewish Cemetery; c. Yanivs'kyi Christian Cemetery; d. Jewish Hospital; e. St. Anna's School; f. Invalidenhaus; g. Shelter for the Poor, the Albertine Brothers' Foundation; h. Execution Mount. Center For Urban History, Lviv.

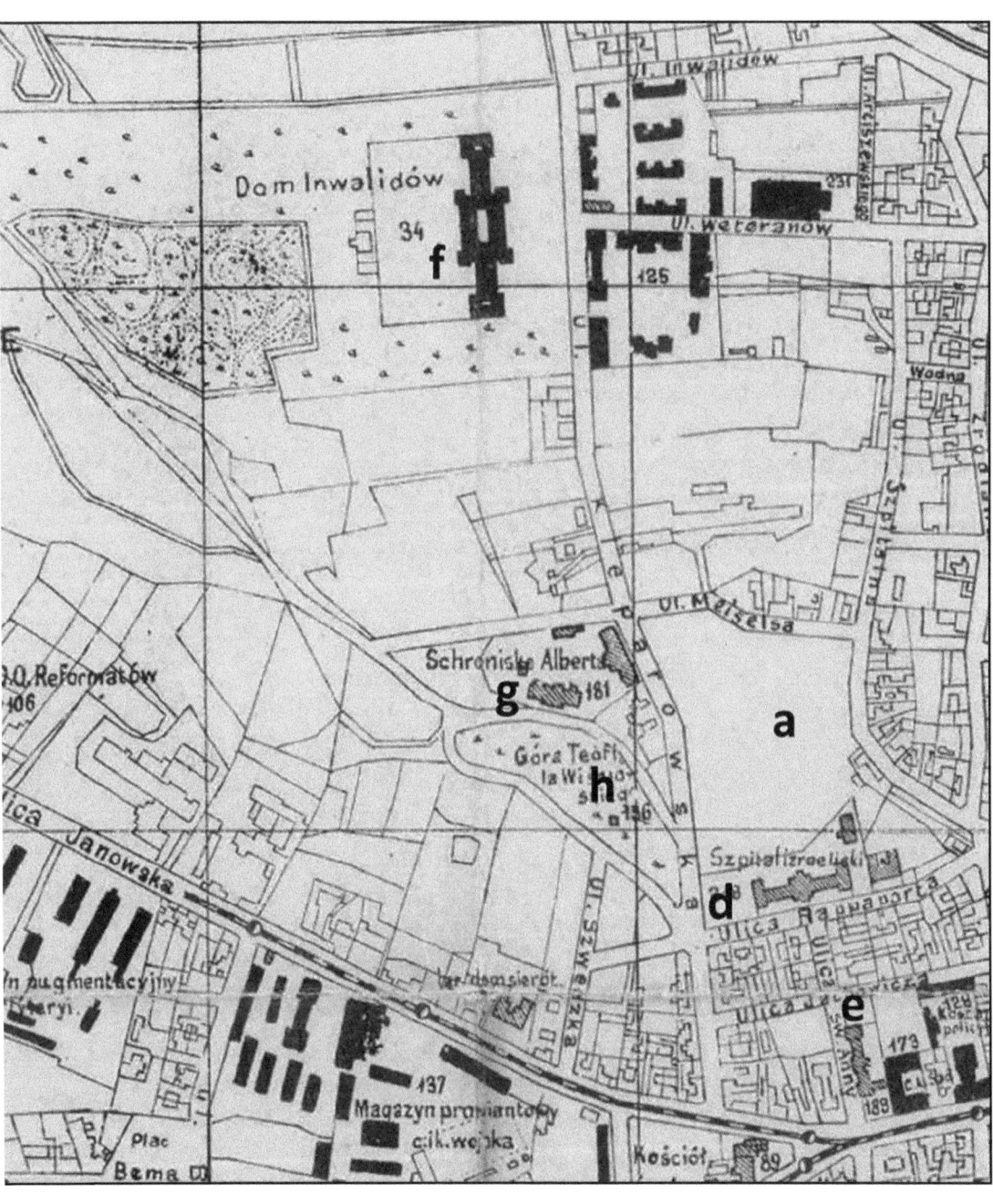

These disagreeable conditions, however, came to an end when a cholera epidemic broke out, and in August 1855 the Old Cemetery was closed (fig. 3.3). Most of the old hospital was demolished in 1902, and only the wing for the incurable remained (figs. 3.4 and 3.5).[8]

The Old People's House, located on the same plot and founded by Israel Taubes and Lazar Rubinstein in 1842, and initially housing sixty patients, was far superior.[9] Subsidized in 1880 by the banker Jakub Stroh, Jakub Klarfeld, Szaja Abraham Buber, and Salomon Ber Berger, the building was extended northwards by the architect Maurycy (Mojżesz Dawid) Silberstein (1857–1912) in 1887 and further enlarged by the architect Antoni Rudolf Fleischl (1862–1921) in 1894; by 1899, it boasted seventy-five beds. In 1903, when the new Jewish Hospital was completed, the Old People's House became part of the new institution.[10] On the corner of Szpitalna (present Bazarna) and Rappaport Streets was Beis Oylem Shul (Cemetery Synagogue), which was run by the suburban burial society (*ḥevra kadisha*).[11] This synagogue dated back to the seventeenth century, a women's gallery was added in 1830, and it was named Moshav Zekenim (the Old People's House) Synagogue after the Old Cemetery was closed.[12]

The improvement of Jewish health care as a result of the creation of the new Jewish Hospital in 1903 became evident in the Kraków suburb (from 1789 the 2nd District of greater Lviv) and became part and parcel of the city's growth and civic advancement (fig. 3.4). A new cemetery, modelled on European and imperial Austrian ones—that is, landscaped—was established in 1855. The old and the new Jewish cemeteries, 1,500 meters apart, were connected by Złota (now Zolota) Street. The Christian communal Janowski (Yanivs'kyi) Cemetery was constructed next to the New Jewish Cemetery in 1888. An enormous Invalidenhaus (home for disabled veterans), supported by the emperor Franz Joseph I, was built in 1855–1860 at Kleparowska (now Kleparivs'ka) Street to the hospital's west. On the corner of Złota and Kleparowska Streets was the Scharfrichtungs Wohnung (Hangman's Quarters); higher up, at top of Execution Mount (Góra Stracenia) were the gallows. In 1894, the city built a monument on Execution Mount to Teofil Wiśniowski (1805–1847) and Józef Kapuściński (1818–1847), participants in the 1846 Kraków Uprising, who were hanged there. In 1892–1896, the Hangman's Quarters gave way to the Shelter for the Poor (paid for and run by the Albertine Brothers' Foundation). Thus, benevolence was at the heart of the city's development.

---

8   Bałaban, "Szpital żydowski," 4; Henryk Mehrer, *Szpital lwowskiej gminy wyznaniowej izraelickiej fundacyi Maurycego Lazarusa* (Lwów: Szpital Lwowskiej Gminy Wyzn. Izraelickiej, 1906), 14–18.
9   Mehrer, *Szpital lwowskiej gminy*, 32.
10 Yurii Biriuliov, *Yevreis'ka arkhitekturna spadshchyna L'vova* (Lviv: Vydavnytstvo Staroho Leva, 2022), 92–93.
11 *Ḥevra kadisha* (Aramaic: Holy society)—the name of traditional Jewish religious associations; commonly applied to the association responsible for performing funerary ceremonies and cemetery maintenance (*ḥevra kadisha gmilat ḥesed shel emet*). In Lviv, the *Ḥevra kadisha* was disbanded in 1827 due to its general dysfunction (along with damage to corpses, fees were extortionate, and members of staff were often drunk, etc.) See Mehrer, *Szpital lwowskiej gminy*, 24.
12 Biriuliov, *Yevreis'ka arkhitekturna spadshchyna*, 41–42.

The foundation, design, construction, and decoration of the Lazarus Jewish Hospital

The new Jewish Hospital building was designed and constructed according to the directions of the donor Maurycy Lazarus, the director of Galician Mortgage Bank and a chairman of the Hospital Council from 1880. He and his wife, Róża, provided three hundred thousand crowns in funds.[13] The new hospital was built close to the old one, west of the Old People's House, on a plot granted by the Jewish community. It was largely completed by the autumn of 1902, and on June 7, 1903, it was opened with great solemnity and transferred for its upkeep to the Jewish Community Council, which was represented by its President Dr. Emil Byk (1845–1906).[14]

Fundamentally, the new hospital was (and still is) a two-story building with a tall basement. Its left (western) wing was assigned to women, and its right (eastern) wing was assigned to men. The ground floor above the basement was for internal medicine (figs. 3.6 and 3.7). Outpatient clinics, their offices, and a shared waiting room were also located on the ground floor, on the right side of the staircase. The registration office, the hospital's administration office, and conference room were on the left (fig. 3.6). The ground floor also housed two rooms for an on-call doctor, as well as a biochemistry laboratory. The surgery department with two operating rooms and the sterilizing room occupied the first floor (fig. 3.8). The basement contained housing for the maintenance personnel and ventilation and low-pressure steam heating systems. The linen, dishes, and equipment storerooms were in the attic.

The hospital included forty-eight rooms for one hundred patients. The rooms were designed for one, two, three, and up to ten patients (fig. 3.9), with every room fitted with a marble basin with cold and hot water. Rooms with one (fig. 3.10), two, or three beds were for those who could pay. Toilets and baths were grouped nearby the staircase on each floor in both wings. The hospital had central water heating, gas lighting, drinking water for everyone, and a boiled water supply for operating rooms. On the ground floor of the eastern wing, the founders had provided, at their own expense, a synagogue (see fig. 4.9 in chapter 4). Two auxiliary buildings housed a kitchen that conformed to the most recent advances in food hygiene (fig. 3.11) and a steam laundry complete with disinfection room (fig. 3.12).

The hospital served Jews and non-Jews alike. The needy Jews of Lviv were treated free of charge, while those from elsewhere in the province paid two, four, or eight crowns per

---

13 Henryk Feuerstein, "Lazarus, życie i czyny lwowskiego filantropa," in *Almanach żydowski wydany przez Hermana Stachla, zawierający szereg artykułów wybitnych literatów, polityków i publicystów oraz życiorysy czołowych postaci Małopolski Wschodniej* (Lwów: Kultura i sztuka, 1937), 216. Józef Wiczkowski, *Lwów, jego rozwój i stan kulturalny oraz przewodnik po mieście* (Lwów: Wydział gospodarczy X. zjazdu lekarzy i przyrodników polskich, oraz reprezentacji m. Lwowa, 1907), 477. Another newspaper account, celebrating Maurycy Lazarus's seventieth jubilee, estimates the cost of the hospital as exceeding six hundred thousand crowns; "Kronika," *Kurjer lwowski* 269 (October 25, 1902): 4. The higher estimate probably included donations for the hospital's maintenance.
14 "Szpital izraelicki fundacji Maurycego Lazarusa," *Gazeta lwowska* 130 (June 9, 1903): 4.

day, depending on "class" of service. In 1907, 655 men and 489 women were treated. Outpatient services were provided to ten thousand Jews and 2,500 Roman and Greek Catholics. Besides these, seventy older members of the Jewish community lived in the Old People's House.[15]

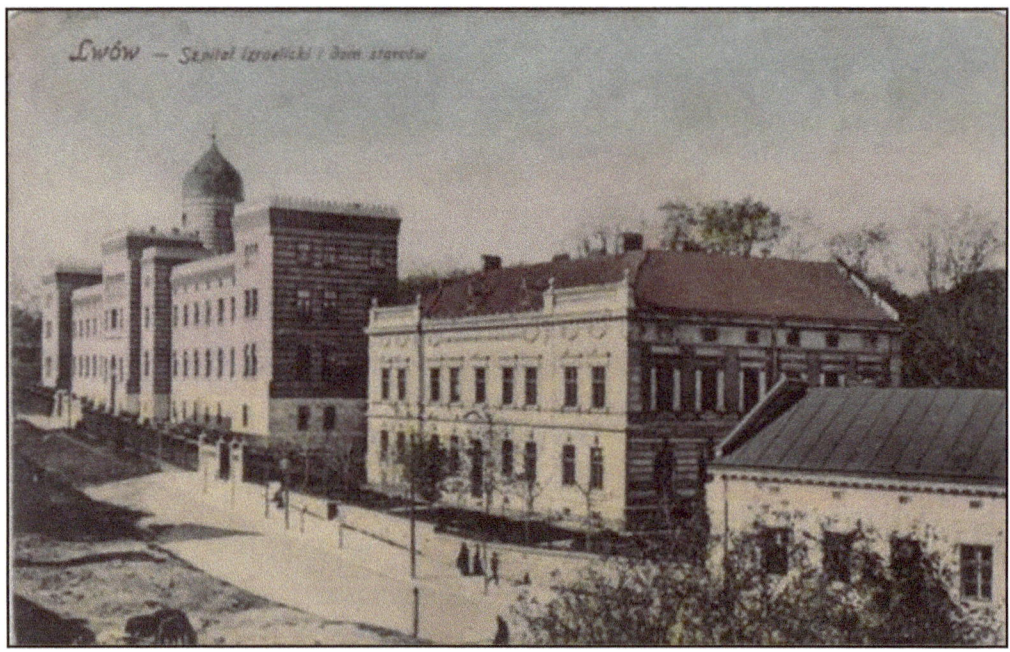

Figure 3.5. The Jewish Hospital (left), the Old People's House (center), and the wing for incurable (right), view from southeast, ca. 1903. Postcard. Courtesy František Bányai.

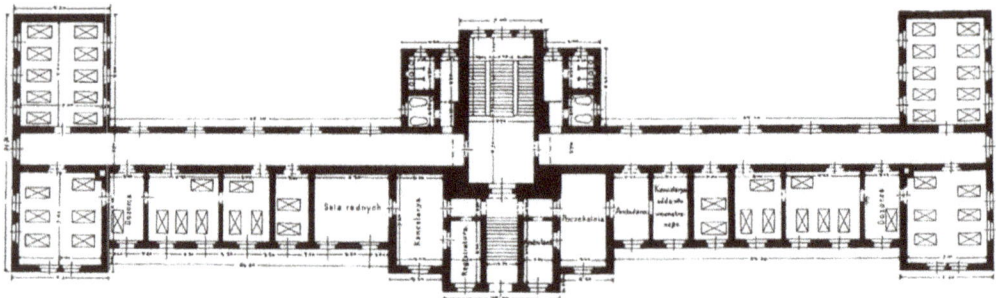

Figure 3.6. The Jewish Hospital, the ground floor plan, 1899, architect Kazimierz Mokłowski. DALO, fond 2, op. 1, spr. 3069, f. 26. Jakub Lewicki, *Między tradycją a nowoczesnością: Architektura Lwowa lat 1893-1918* (Warsaw: Neriton, 2021), 92.

---

15 Wiczkowski, *Lwów*, 477.

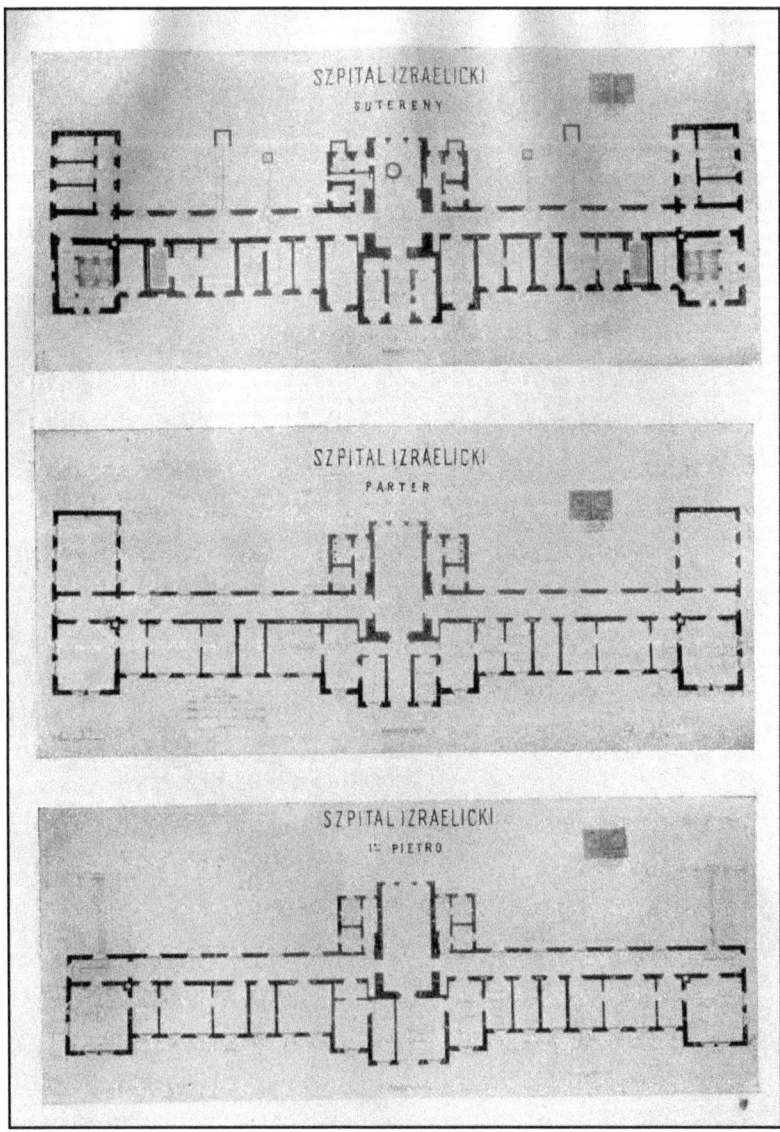

Figure 3.7. The Jewish Hospital, floor plans, 1898. Mehrer, *Szpital lwowskiej gminy*, 53.

As originally designed, built, and preserved, the hospital's new and remarkable building faces Rappaport Street, while its rear looks over the ancient cemetery,[16] which was already closed in 1855 and sunken in greenery (figs. 3.2 and 3.5). The building's symmetry, slightly distorted by the street's rise, corresponds to the division between male and female patients (fig. 3.13). The edifice is flanked by three-story wings and accentuated by a towering central avant-corps crowned with a tall drum, above which is a pointed dome covered with brown,

---

16 The Old Jewish Cemetery was destroyed during and after World War II.

ocher, blue, and green glazed ceramic tiles,[17] topped, in turn, with a Star of David (missing since World War II). The wings were only the ground-floor high on the rear (northern) side of the building because the internal medicine department demanded twenty beds more than the surgery.[18] The flat roofs of these ground-floor northern protrusions were landscaped to serve as fenced terraces for convalescent patients (fig. 3.14). With some hyperbole, a report on the nearly finished hospital compares these first-floor terraces to the one of the Seven Wonders of the World, the hanging gardens of Babylon, to be precise.[19]

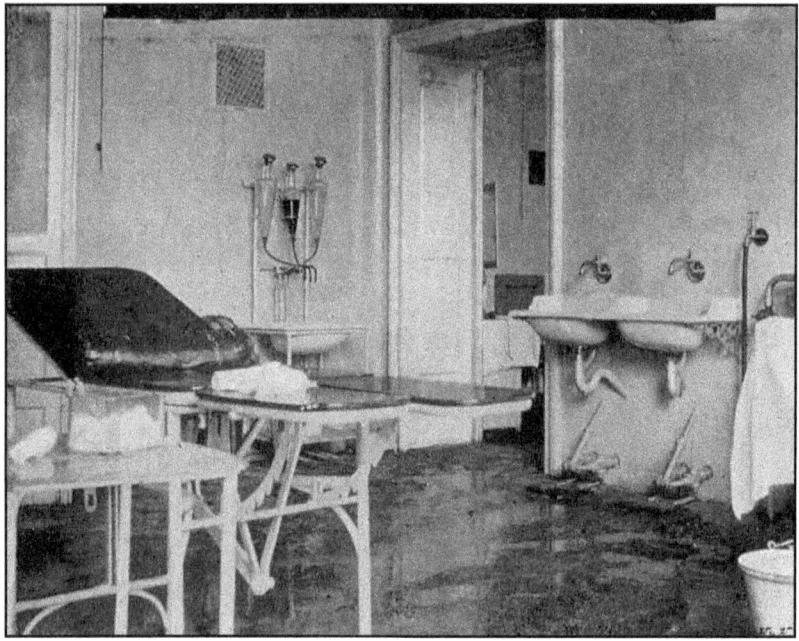

Figure 3.8. The Jewish Hospital, operating room. Mehrer, *Szpital lwowskiej gminy*, 29.

The façade is of red and yellow brick, arranged in horizontal strips and Stars of David. The hospital's elevations are pierced with pointed, ogee, horseshoe-shaped, cusped, round, and rectangular openings. The stalactite-shaped crowning cornices support a Moresque openwork embattlement screening a low-pitched roof. The street façade bore signage in Polish: Szpital Izraelicki Fundacyi Maurycego Lazarusa (Maurycy Lazarus Foundation Israelite Hospital), now obliterated. The entire compound was surrounded by an openwork redbrick wall designed in 1902 by the architect Władysław Godowski (1842–1910).

---

17 Andrii Klimashevs'kyi ed., *Keramichnyi kod Ivana Levyns'koho v estetychnomu vymiri ukraintsia XIX – pochatku XX st.* (Lviv: Rarytety Ukrainy, 2020), 92–93. The cupola's tiles are flat "beavertails" that are customarily used on steep roofs.
18 Mehrer, *Szpital lwowskiej gminy*, 12.
19 Bałaban, "Szpital żydowski," 4.

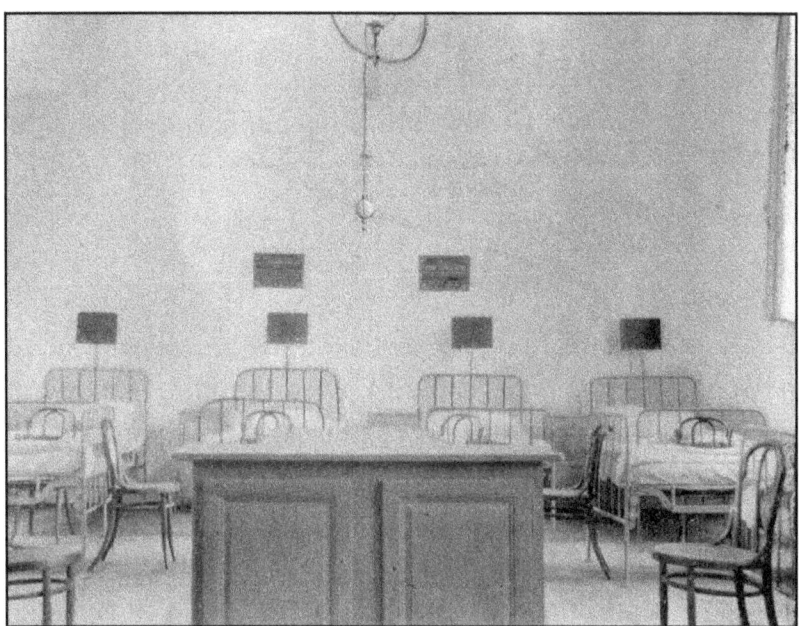

Figure 3.9. The Jewish Hospital, patient room. Mehrer, *Szpital lwowskiej gminy*, 23.

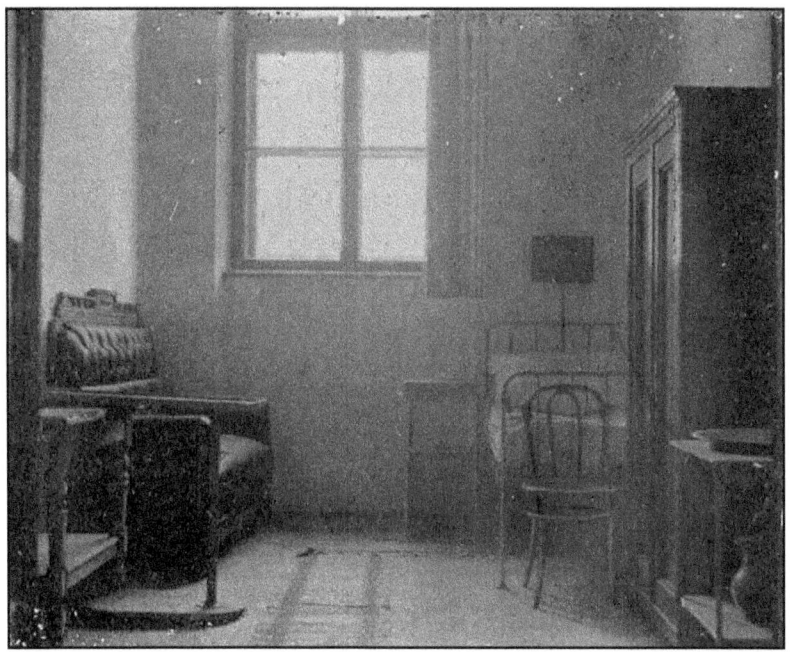

Figure 3.10. The Jewish Hospital, first-class room. Mehrer, *Szpital lwowskiej gminy*, 25.

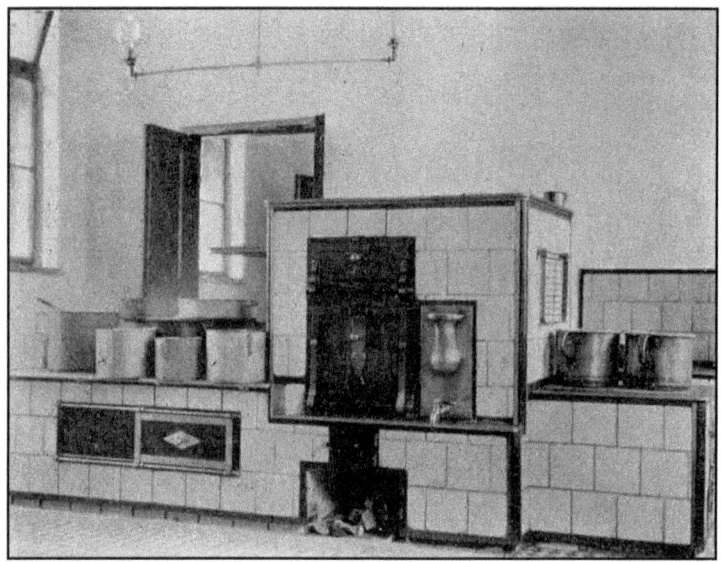

Figure 3.11. The Jewish Hospital, kitchen. Mehrer, *Szpital lwowskiej gminy*, 43.

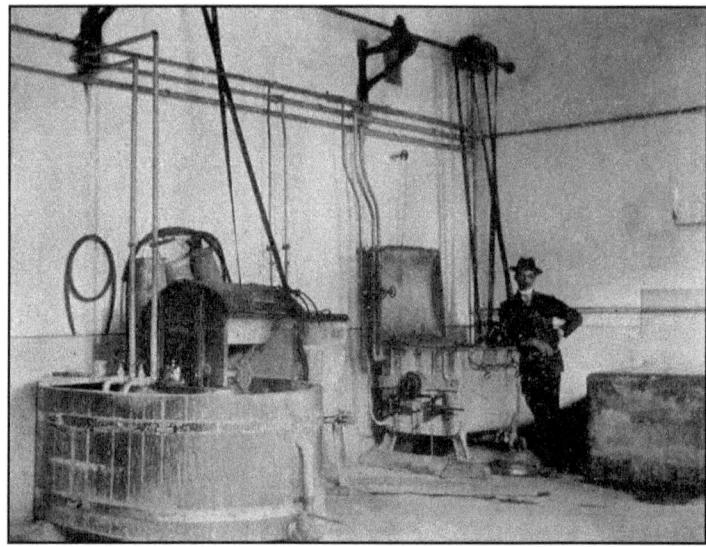

Figure 3.12. The Jewish Hospital, laundry. Mehrer, *Szpital lwowskiej gminy*, 45.

The hospital's interior layout uses space very efficiently and has a central staircase (fig. 3.6). Most rooms face Rappaport Street on the south, while the corridor faces the north backyard (fig. 3.15). This orientation facilitated natural draught ventilation of the rooms, as air quality and getting enough sunlight were at the forefront of health care at that time. The corridors were also fitted with ducts that circulated warm air from the basement installation to every room. Cold air was originally drawn from two tanks in the garden. Inside the tanks, filters and water sprays purified the air, and it was then moved to four basement chambers, where it was heated to +15°C (59°F), +20°C (68°F), or +25°C

(77°F), depending on requirements. From these chambers, the air was distributed around the building, and ultimately it was vented through the chimneys. This heating system was designed for the minimal exterior temperature, –25°C (–13°F), and there were radiators in every room.

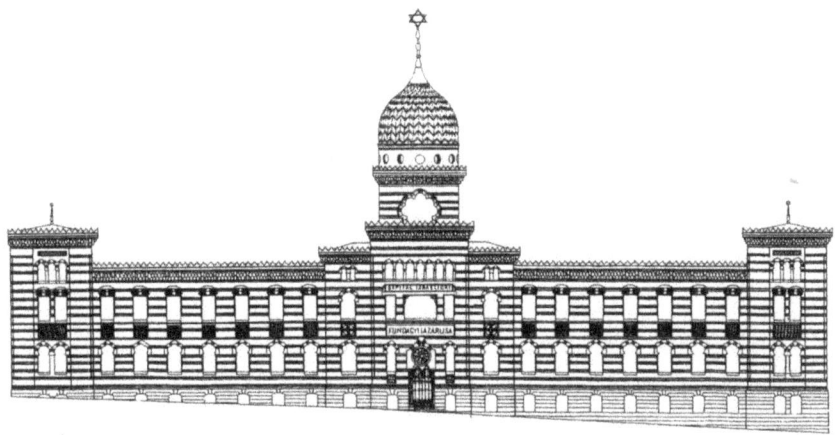

Figure 3.13. The Jewish Hospital, southern facade, 1899; architect Kazimierz Mokłowski. DALO, fond. 2, op. 1, spr. 3069, f. 23. Lewicki, *Między tradycją a nowoczesnością: Architektura Lwowa lat 1893-1918*, 92.

The hospital interior was airy and clean, with whitewashed walls. The main interior embellishment was the vestibule decorated in a "pure Moorish style" by the Maurycy (Yitzhak Moshe, 1858–1932) and Isidor (Eisig) Fleck brothers, a firm renowned for its work on numerous public buildings and synagogues.[20] In the boardroom was a large portrait of Maurycy Lazarus sitting in an armchair, painted in 1902 by the emerging artist Wilhelm Wachtel (1875–1952;[21] figs. 3.16 and 3.17).[22] At the proposal of the Jewish Community Council,[23] the main staircase received a Moresque-framed niche containing a marble bust of the founder (fig. 3.18) by the well-known Polish sculptor Antoni Popiel (1865–1910). Urban folklore has it that the 1903 bust of Lazarus was preserved under Soviet rule, since it

---

20 Galina Glembotskaya, *Khudozhniki-evrei L'vova pervoi poloviny XX veka: Zhizn', tvorchestvo, sud'ba* (Lviv: Stavropigion, 2015), 390–391. Maurycy Fleck was the father of Ludwik Fleck (1896–1962), a microbiologist who developed the first system of historical philosophy and sociology of science.
21 Wilhelm Wachtel (1875 [Lviv]–1952 [New York]) studied at the School of Fine Arts in Kraków between 1895 and 1898 under Leon Wyczółkowski and Leopold Löffler, and then at the Academy of Fine Arts in Munich under Nikolaus Gysis. He traveled frequently to Vienna, Paris, and Palestine. From 1938, he lived in Habana (Cuba) and the US. Wachtel is known for his portraits, Zionist-inspired scenes of Jewish life in the Diaspora and the Land of Israel, and biblical compositions.
22 This portrait is held in the Borys Voznytsky Lviv National Art Gallery, inv. no Ж-3727. Anastasiia Simferovska, "L'vivs'kyi portret pershoi polovyny XX stolittia: Khudozhnia representatsiia osobystosti," Ph.D. diss., L'vivs'ka Natsional'na Akademiia Mystetstv, 2018, 222, fig. 2.1.32, accessed November 30, 2022, lnam.edu.ua/files/Academy/nauka/specrada/Rozklad/18.10.18/dissertation%20simferovska-compressed.pdf.
23 "Szpital izraelicki fundacji Maurycego Lazarusa," 4.

was creatively attributed by the locals to the Russian surgeon Nikolai Pirogov (1810–1881). In fact, the current bust was installed by the Soviets in 1940 (fig. 3.19) and is a monument to Pirogov (well known from several portraits and photographs), rather than Lazarus, who was photographed and portrayed by the painters Wilhelm Wachtel (fig. 3.17) and Maurycy Trębacz (1861–1941).[24] Unfortunately, I have been unable to locate the original bust of Maurycy Lazarus.[25]

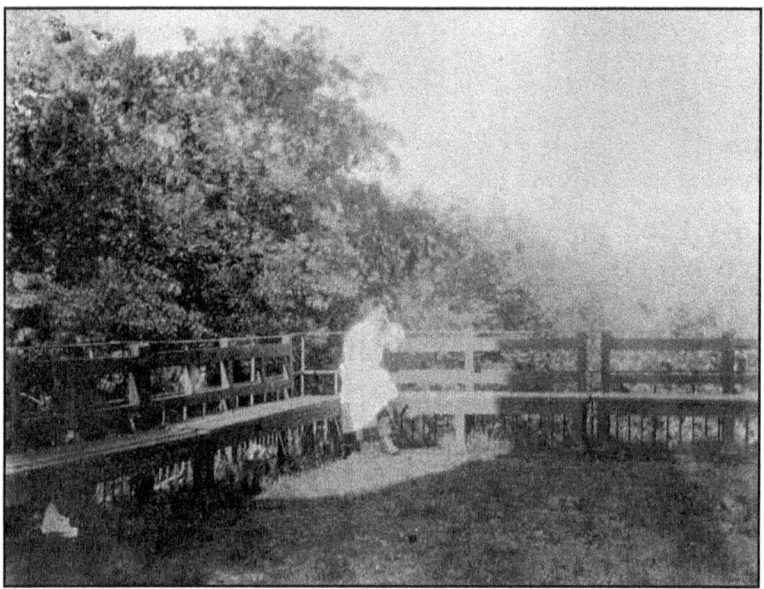

Figure 3.14. The Jewish Hospital, terrace for convalescent patients. Mehrer, *Szpital lwowskiej gminy*, 247.

The architectural style of the Jewish Hospital

Contemporaries identified the hospital's style as Moorish, and in 1916 it was described as "Romanesque oriental."[26] These definitions, however, do not capture its local and historical usage.

Enlightened Jewish society was behind the nineteenth-century Moorish Revival style in synagogue architecture. The perception that Jews experienced a "Golden Age" under the Moors in medieval Spain owed much to the Ashkenazi intellectuals Abraham Geiger (1810–1874) and Heinrich Graetz (1817–1871). The Jewish life that flourished in Muslim

---

24 Portraits of Maurycy Lazarus are stored at the Borys Voznytsky Lviv National Art Gallery and the Jewish Historical Institute in Warsaw.
25 On the removal of the bust see Biriuliov, *Yevreis'ka arkhitekturna spadshchyna*, 88. I am profoundly grateful to Lviv art historians Ihor Siomochkin and Anna Bantsekova for finding archival materials located in the Borys Voznytsky Lviv National Art Gallery for me.
26 Bałaban, "Szpital żydowski," 4; Josef Piotrowski, *Lemberg: Handbuch für Kunstliebhaber u. Reisende* (Lwów: H. Altenberg, G. Seyfarth, E. Wende & Co, 1916), 144.

Spain was, for these writers, defined by social consolidation, cultural openness, progress in philosophy and the arts, and integration with the host society,[27] and it served as a model for proponents of Reform Judaism and Jewish emancipation in Prussia.

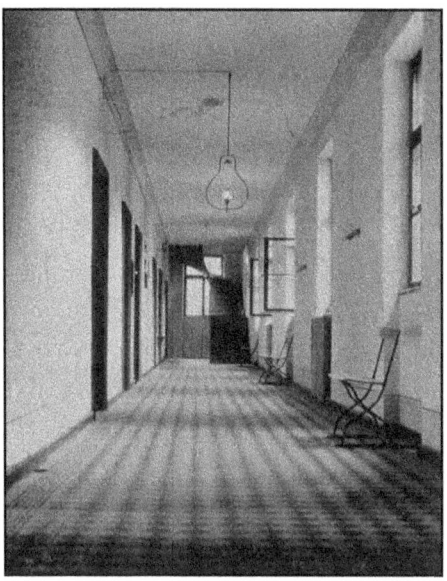

Figure 3.15. The Jewish Hospital, corridor. Mehrer, *Szpital lwowskiej gminy*, 21.

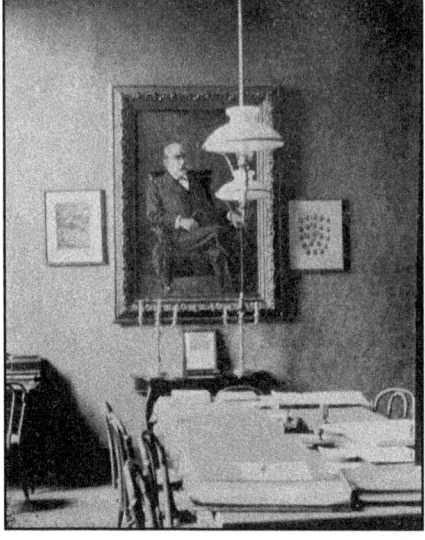

Figure 3.16. The Jewish Hospital, conference room. Mehrer, *Szpital lwowskiej gminy*, 19.

---

27 Ismar Schorsch, "The Myth of Sephardic Supremacy," *Leo Baeck Institute Year Book* 34, no. 1 (January 1989): 47, https://doi.org/10.1093/leobaeck/34.1.47.

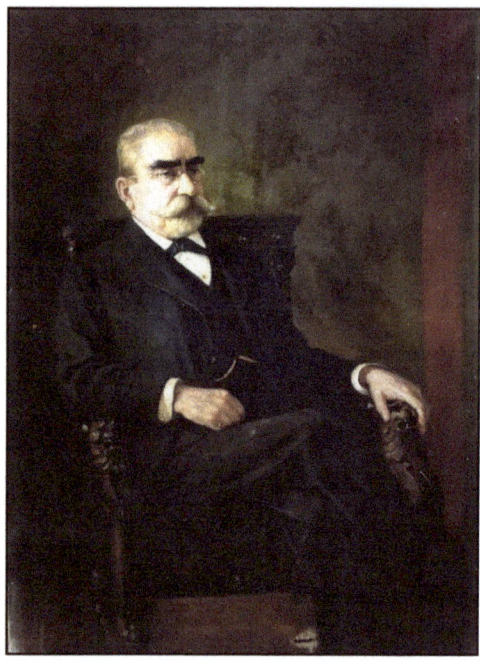

Figure 3.17. Portrait of Maurycy Lazarus by Wilhelm Wachtel, 1902. Oil on canvas. Borys Voznytsky Lviv National Art Gallery.

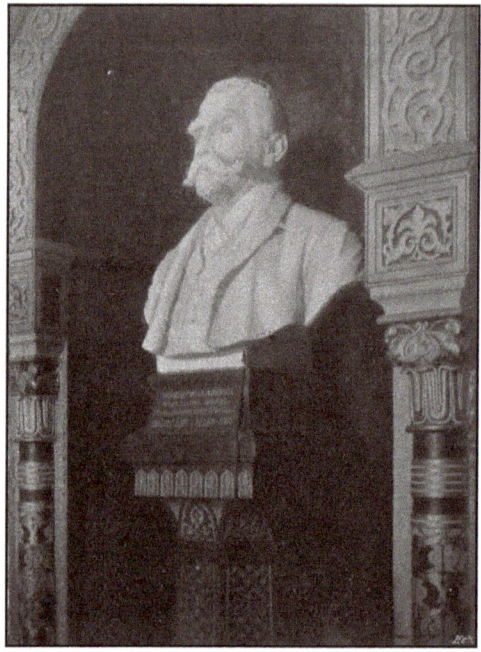

Figure 3.18. The Jewish Hospital, bust of Maurycy Lazarus by sculptor Antoni Popiel. Mehrer, *Szpital lwowskiej gminy*, 15.

A combination of Romanesque and Moorish influences at times had been in vogue in the Habsburg lands. First employed by the Viennese architects Ludwig Förster (1797–1863) and Theophilus Hansen (1813–1891) in Baron Adolf Pereira's villa in 1847, it evoked both the "romance" of the Orient and Pereira's Sephardic roots.[28] After the 1848 "Spring of Nations," Förster and Hansen added other styles to the Romanesque and Byzantine, mostly borrowed from the empire's historical domains such as Iberian, Italian, German, and Balkan lands. This replaced the stern neoclassicism of the *Vormärz* (the period before the March Revolution of 1848), which became retrospectively associated with Metternich's repressive regime. In much later literature, this novel style received the name Romantic Historicism. However, Hansen pretentiously called it Viennese Renaissance,[29] thereby emphasizing its political significance rather than its Italianate component.

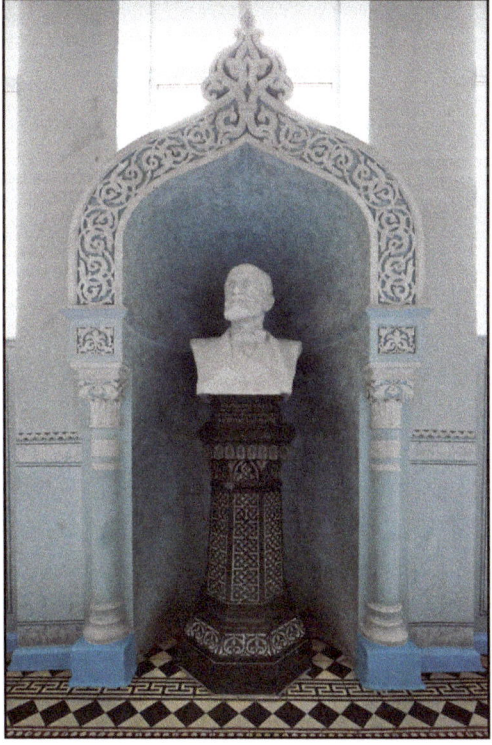

Figure 3.19. Bust of Nikolai Pirogov replacing the original bust of Lazarus. Photo Yulia Korytska-Holub, 2023.

---

28 Ludwig Förster, "Die Baron Pereira'sche Willa aus der Herrschaft Königstetten im Tullnerboden nächst Wien," *Allgemeine Bauzeitung* (1849): 107.
29 Stefan Muthesius, "Renate Wagner-Rieger and Mara Reissenberg, *Theophil von Hansen* (Die Wiener Ringstrasse, Bild einer Epoche, vol. 4, Section VIII) (Wiesbaden, 1980)," *Journal of the Society of Architectural Historians* 42, no. 1 (1983): 80–81.

Due to its synthetic nature, Viennese Renaissance style was easily adapted to suit the identities of the architects' diverse clientele. In the late 1840s and 1850s, Förster and Hansen applied this style to Orthodox and Protestant churches, such as the Greek Orthodox Church in Vienna I (1857) and the Evangelical Church in Gumpendorf, Vienna VI (1849); an all-purpose chapel at the Lviv Invalidenhaus (1855–1860); synagogues in Tempelgasse, Vienna II (1856–58) and Dohány Street, Budapest (1854–1859); and such monumental imperial projects as the Waffenmuseum in Vienna (1852–1856) and the Invalidenhaus in Lviv (fig. 3.20).

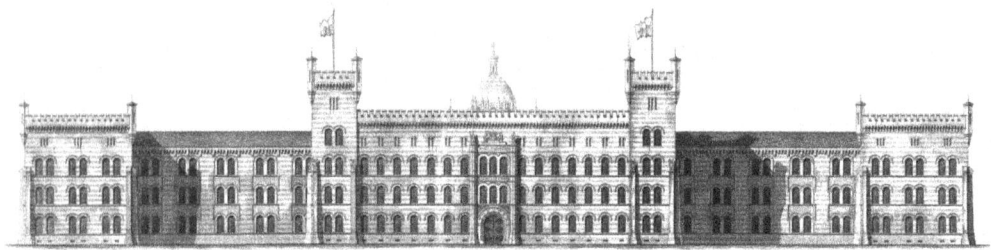

Figure 3.20. Invalidenhaus in Lviv, architect Theophilus Hansen, 1855. "Das k.k. Invalidenhaus in Lemberg," *Allgemeine Bauzeitung*, no. 25 (1860), plate 338.

It became the signature of an empire that stretched from East to West, one in which multiple religions harmoniously coexisted under an enlightened liberal regime, and where the emperor cared about the well-being of his subjects.[30]

The Viennese Renaissance was also applied to Ukrainian community buildings. The Ruthenian National Institute in Lviv (Narodnyi Dim, 1851–1864) was constructed along these lines after a design by Wilhelm Schmidt.[31] The architect was born in the German colony of Weinbergen, otherwise known as the Lviv suburb of Winniki (now Vynnyky), and worked in the Galician metropolis.[32] The Trinitarian Monastery, which once stood on the Ruthenian Institute's plot, was converted into Lviv University by Emperor Joseph II, but burned down during the revolutionary events of 1848. Emperor Franz Joseph I "rewarded" the Ruthenian community of Lviv with this parcel of land for their loyalty during that turbulent year. The emperor laid the cornerstone of the future institute and a church during a visit to Lviv in 1851.[33] Thus, the entire project was rich in imperial significance. However, the exterior of the Ruthenian National Institute was far less expressive than the examples of Romantic Historicism built by Viennese architects, since Schmidt had worked for decades

---

30 Sergey R. Kravtsov, "Jewish Identities in Synagogue Architecture of Galicia and Bukovina," *Ars Judaica* 6 (2010): 94.
31 Volodymyr Vuitsyk, "Narodnyi Dim u L'vovi," in *Visnyk instytutu "Ukrzakhidproektrestavratsia,"* vol. 14 (Lviv: Ukrzakhidproektrestavratsia, 2004), 165. The building was constructed under the supervision of the young architect Sylwester Hawryszkiewicz (1833–1911).
32 Stanisław Łoza, *Słownik architektów i budowniczych Polaków oraz cudzoziemców w Polsce pracujących* (Warsaw: Kasa im. Mianowskiego Instytutu Popierania Nauki, 1931), 301.
33 Prokopovych, *Habsburg Lemberg*, 146–149.

in provincial Lviv and was an adept of "Biedermeier Classicism."[34] Unlike its polychrome brick analogues, the institute was plastered in simple fashion—an approach that would have been more appropriate in downtown Lviv.

In the "Jewish" versions of the new style—the synagogues of Vienna and Pest—Förster further developed its specifically Jewish elements. He introduced the idea of Solomon's Temple, focusing particularly on that building's tripartite division, thereby charging his work with additional authority.[35] He never included domes or cupolas in synagogues, an element alien to the Temple of Jerusalem as described in the Bible or Mishnah.[36] A cupola was proposed by the prominent German architect Gottfried Semper (1803–1879), who argued that in the Dresden New Synagogue it represented "the seven heavens of the Old Testament"[37]—although the "seven heavens" are actually mentioned for the first time in Judaism in the Babylonian Talmud (Chagigah 12b).[38] This meaning for cupolas was later implied by Julian Zachariewicz (1837–1898), a rising Vienna-educated architect, in his design for the Progressive Synagogue in Chernivtsi (German: Czernowitz, 1873–78, fig. 3.21). In his Progressive Synagogue (Lviv) project in the 1890s, the cupola imaged an open sky and hence the Tempel's courtyard. Maurycy Lazarus was aware of this architectural sophistication, as he headed the building committee to which Zachariewicz had presented his project.[39] The Chernivtsi and Lviv Progressive Synagogues also employed domes to signify that there was a Jewish presence in the city that extended beyond the old Jewish quarters. In the case of the Jewish Hospital, the dome, quite similar in its "Oriental" silhouette to that of the Progressive Synagogue of Chernivtsi, was part of a secular Jewish building. While the hospital was not a synagogue, its lofty dome was appropriate: it pointed to the heavenly, and not the terrestrial, sphere.

According to Förster and Hansen, brick façades evoked archeological finds in the Middle East and Byzantium. In the second half of the nineteenth century, this idea merged with the so-called Brick Gothic and was regarded as an efficient and durable solution to building schools, hospitals, and prisons. The architect Juliusz Hochberger (1840–1905) used brick cladding in Lviv's St. Anna's School (figs. 3.22 and 3.23), constructed in 1884 on the corner of St. Anna (now Leontovycha) Street, which runs from Kazimierzowska (now Horodotska) thoroughfare in the direction of the hospital.[40] While broadly typical of

---

34 Jurij Biriulow, *Rzeźba lwowska od połowy XVIII wieku do 1939 roku* (Warsaw: Neriton, 2007), 26–27.
35 Ludwig Förster, "Das israelitische Bethhaus in der Wiener Vorstadt Leopoldstadt," *Allgemeine Bauzeitung* (1859): 14.
36 The Mishnah (Heb.: "study by repetition") is the earlier part of the Talmud, a compendium of the Oral Torah written down in Palestine in about 200 CE. "Mishnah" can also refer to a paragraph or verse from the tractates of the Mishnah. The Mishnaic treatise Middot includes a detailed description of the Herodian Temple.
37 Gottfried Semper, "Die Synagoge zu Dresden," *Allgemeine Bauzeitung* 12 (1847): 127.
38 Babylonian Talmud (Heb.: "Instruction") is the central text of Rabbinic Judaism, which comprises the Mishnah and the Gemara (Aramaic: "Mastery, completion"), written ca. 500 CE. The Gemara is a commentary on the Mishnah and related writings.
39 "Sprawozdanie ze zgromadzenia odb. d. 29 stycznia r.b.," *Czasopismo techniczne* 14, no. 5 (1896): 58.
40 In 1884, St. Anna Street was a dead-end street, not connected to Rappaport Street.

European schools and Catholic structures, it also drew on Romantic Historicism by way of materials, ornament, and fenestration.

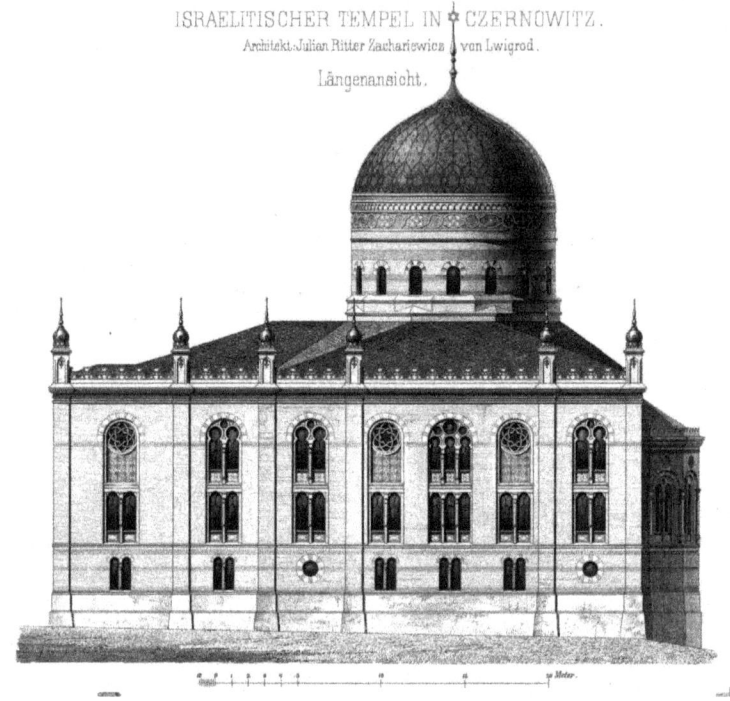

Figure 3.21. Progressive Synagogue in Chernivtsi, architect Julian Zachariewicz, 1873–1878, southern façade. Julian Zachariewicz, "Israelitischer Tempel in Czernowitz," *Allgemeine Bauzeitung*, no. 47 (1882), plate 29.

Hochberger, who headed the City Building Administration between 1872 and 1905 and designed many significant buildings in the Galician metropolis, favored architectural coherence in the urban environment. He continued the Romantic Historicism towards the west of the Old Cemetery and the future hospital on the opposite side of Kleparowska Street. In 1892–1896, he built the Shelter for the Poor there (fig. 3.24).[41] This single-story compound featured a red and yellow brick façade with Romanesque Revival fenestration, matching St. Anna's School and the Invalidenhaus.[42]

Thus, the Jewish Hospital, with its impressive southern façade and brickwork wall, was a new stage in a long architectural and urban process, a nexus between the Invalidenhaus and the Shelter for the Poor on Kleparowska Street to its west and St. Anna's School to its south. From the outset, then, the hospital was designed with aesthetic consistency in mind. This urban strategy, as will be shown, was continued in the same vicinity after the inauguration of the hospital's main building.

---

41 The foundation was established by Albert Chmielowski (1845–1916), a Polish nobleman, painter, and disabled veteran of the 1863 uprising. Pope John Paul II canonized Chmielowski in 1989.
42 Yurii Biriuliov, *Lwów: Ilustrowany przewodnik* (Lviv: Centrum Europy, 2003), 144.

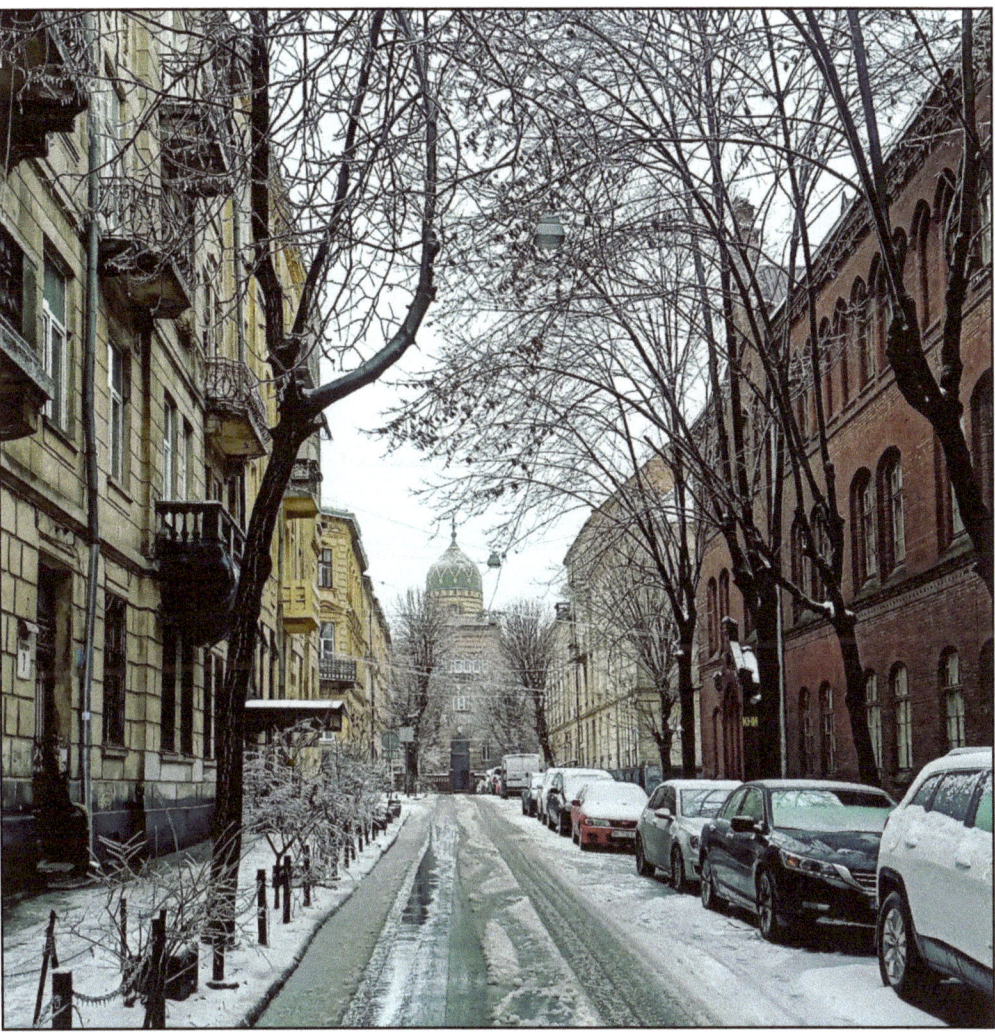

Figure 3.22. The Jewish Hospital and St. Anna's School (on the right), by architect Juliusz Hochberger, northern extension by firm of Michał Ulam. View from the south. Photo g_vikki, posted on Facebook, November 2022.

The building of a new hospital did not meet any resistance since it was built on the plot that had belonged to the Jewish community for five centuries. The new Jewish visibility in the overwhelmingly Christian cityscape was not the result of a new acquisition, as was the case, for instance, with the Progressive Synagogue in the old marketplace, which increasingly troubled conservative Catholics.[43] In fact, the Jewish Hospital was a welcome addition to the city's health care infrastructure.

Romantic Historicism was not fashionable for the whole of the mid-nineteenth century. In the 1860s, it gave way to so-called Strict Historicism during the construction of the Vienna Ring Road that replaced the city's fortifications. The new architecture married

---

43 Cf. Jan Sas-Zubrzycki, *Zabytki miasta Lwowa* (Lwów: Nakładem autora, 1928), 6.

historical forms to function. For example, August Sicard von Sicardsburg, Eduard van der Nüll, and Josef Hlávka built the Vienna State Opera (1861–1869) in the Renaissance Revival style in order to evoke the origins of opera; Theophilus Hansen designed the Austrian Parliament Building (1874–1883) in the Greek Revival because democracy was born in ancient Athens; Friedrich Schmidt's work borrowed Flemish and Brabant Gothic for the Viennese Townhall (1872–1883) in order to refer to fair urban self-government. The Moorish Revival remained, however, the convention for Jewish constructions in Lviv until the outbreak of World War I.[44]

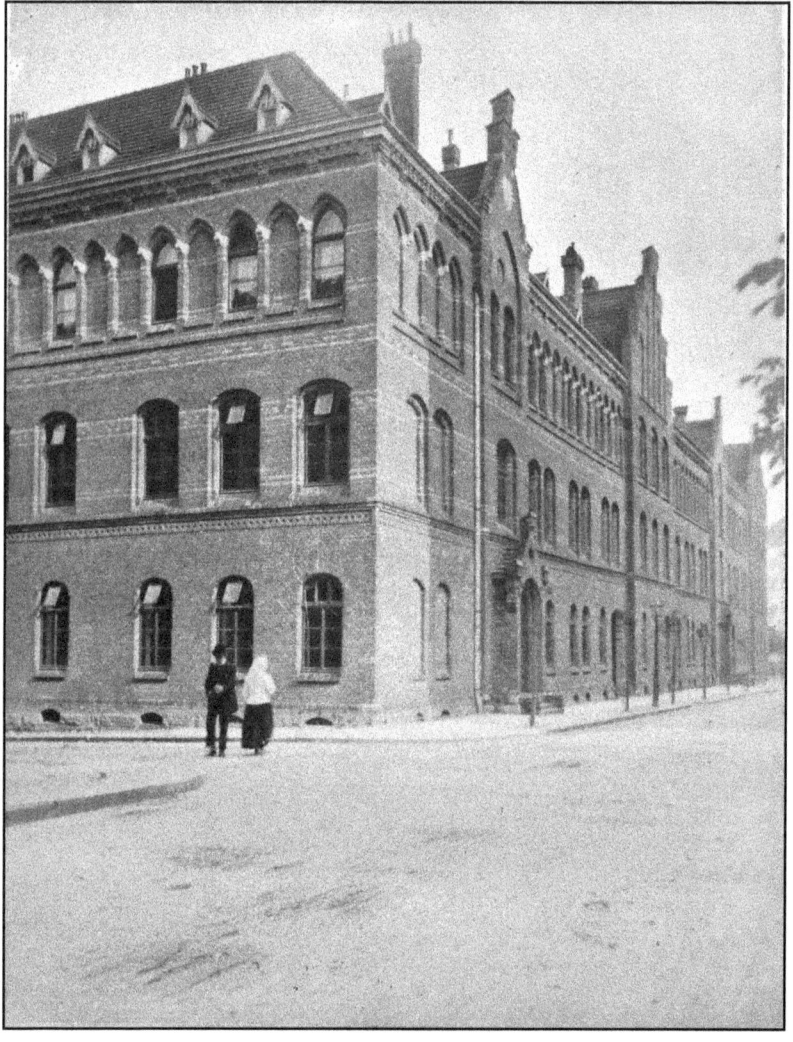

Figure 3.23. Extension of St. Anna's School by firm of Michał Ulam, ca. 1913, view from northwest. *Budowle wykonane w dziesięcioleciu 1903-1913 przez firmę Michał Ulam architekt-budowniczy, Lwów* (Lwów: Unia, 1913), unpaginated.

---

44 Ivan Davidson Kalmar, "Orientalism, the Jews, and Synagogue Architecture," *Jewish Social Studies*, n.s., 7, no. 3 (Spring–Summer, 2001): 69.

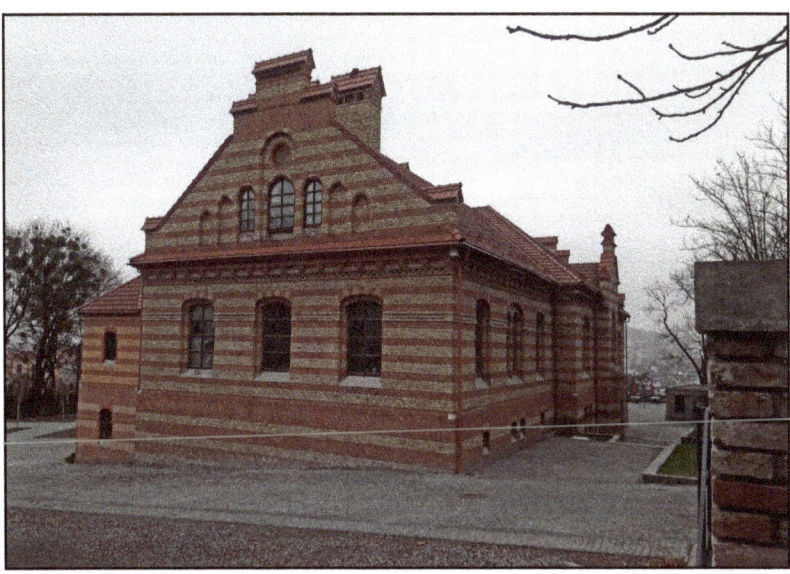

Figure 3.24. Shelter for the Poor of the Albertine Brothers' Foundation on the corner of Kleparivs'ka and Zolota Streets, architect Juliusz Hochberger, 1892–1896. Photo Tetiana Kazantseva, 2024.

By 1900, the assimilated Jews of Vienna turned away from the Moorish Revival and embraced the Romanesque and Gothic, which they considered truly Germanic, as proposed by assimilated architects like Jacob Gartner (1861–1921) and Max Fleischer (1841–1905) for Jewish sacred, secular, and funerary buildings. In Lviv, Julian Zachariewicz advanced an alternative "Jewish style" based on the reconstruction of Ezechiel's vision of the Temple by the French authors Georges Perrot and Charles Chipiez, who combined Egyptian, Assyrian, Phoenician, and Palestinian patterns.[45] Zachariewicz's "forsaken style" challenged the dominance of the "Moorish, Gothic, [and] Romanesque."[46]

Moorish Revival architecture survived, albeit on a smaller scale. Wilhelm Stiassny (1842–1910) used it for the Polish Rite Synagogue in Vienna. Many of his works at the turn of the century, including his protuberant Moorish Revival Jubilee Synagogue in Prague (1905–6), were highly exotic. There are several possible reasons to explain their exuberant otherness. Firstly, Stiassny was a Zionist and wished to assert Jewishness. Secondly, the Jubilee Synagogue was established on the sixtieth anniversary of the emperor's reign, a period which saw Austrian Jews attained full rights, and Romantic Historicism marked the fall of the ancien régime. Though free of Zionist fervor, the Jubilee Orthodox Synagogue in Tarnów (by the architect Władysław Ekielski, 1865–1908) had Moorish Revival features. The Moorish style of the Jewish Hospital should also be seen as a proud manifestation of Jewishness and a jubilee retrospect. Indeed, Lazarus explicitly stated his own desire "to celebrate the fiftieth jubilee of the reign of Franz Joseph I" with the new hospital.[47]

---

45 Charles Chipiez and Georges Perrot, *Le Temple de Jérusalem et la Maison du Bois-Liban restitués d'après Ezéchiel et le Livre des Rois* (Paris: Hachette, 1889).
46 "Sprawozdanie ze zgromadzenia," 58.
47 TsDIAL, fond 701, op. 2, spr. 1559, f. 55. Lazarus formulated his decision to set up the hospital ca. 1898.

The architects of the hospital

Maurycy Lazarus recruited the best contractors in Lviv to implement his ambitious plans.

Ivan Ivanovych Levyns'kyi

Lazarus hired the firm of Ivan Levyns'kyi—known as Jan Lewiński, Master Builder—to work on the hospital (fig. 3.25). An outstanding architect and businessman, Levyns'kyi was born in Dolyna (Polish: Dolina) in 1851. His father, Ivan Levyns'kyi Sr., was a member of the Ukrainian petty gentry and an elementary school principal; his mother, Josefa née Hauser, was from a family of Bavarian colonists in Galicia. Ivan attended an elementary school in Stryi (Polish: Stryj) and the Secondary Technical School (c. k. Wyższa Szkoła Realna) in Lviv. In 1869–1874, he studied at Lviv Technical University,[48] graduated as an architect and engineer, secured a builder's license in 1881, and started his company in partnership with Julian Zachariewicz. At its most successful, the company employed about one thousand workers who worked sixteen-hour days. The firm designed buildings and oversaw their construction. Moreover, they manufactured brick, ceramic, gypsum, concrete, artificial stone, stained glass, wooden doors and windows, and much more. They received the best commissions, including the Opera House, the Georges Hotel, and the new Lviv railway station. Levyns'kyi managed about two hundred construction sites simultaneously. From 1901, he worked as a professor at his alma mater while also running the company.

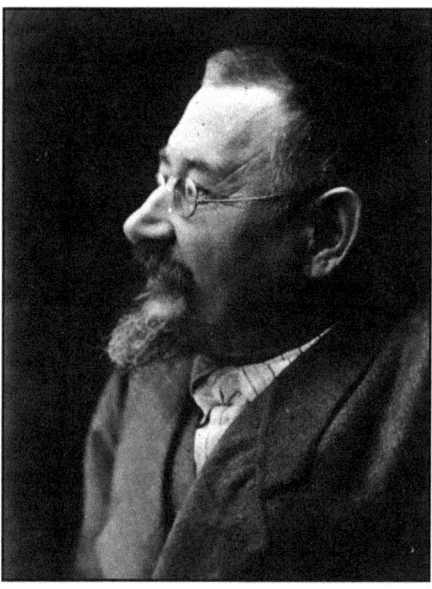

Figure 3.25. Ivan Levyns'sky, 1851–1919. LNNBU.

---

48 The names changed over the years: "Technical Academy" (Polish: "Akademia Techniczna"; German "Technische Akademie") in 1844–77; "Polytechnical School" (Polish: "Szkoła Politechniczna"; German: "Technische Hochschule") in 1877–1914; "Lviv Polytechnic" (Polish: "Politechnika Lwowska") in 1919–39.

A master builder (*budowniczy*)—that is, an engineer, architect, businessman, and pedagogue— Levyns'kyi developed and popularized his own aesthetic. He believed that all buildings could be divided into two categories. In the first, the utilitarian was foremost: such buildings were intended "to give people everything they need for life and culture." The second concerned "monumental" buildings—those that were to capture the state's social, political, religious, and cultural values. These edifices, constructed from the most durable materials, embodied the nation's soul and were to last for the benefit of future generations. Levyn'skyi explained that "the designer decides how much space on the horizontal plane is required to fulfill the building's purpose; simultaneously, he groups the masses and thus erects the edifice above the ground plane." For Levyn'skyi, then, the ground plan was the preserve of master builder; the architect's domain was the elevations, the "aesthetic forms" so crucial for monumental structures.[49]

Due to its reputation and experience, Levyns'ky's firm was hired to oversee the Jewish Hospital's design and construction, as well as source its materials. Most probably, the efficient ground plan of the Jewish Hospital reflects the master builder Levyn'skyi's thought and experience, whereas its "aesthetic forms" were designed by an able architect, who will be introduced in due course. It is likely that materials were supplied by Levyns'kyi's factories,[50] including the brown, ocher, blue, and green glazed ceramic tiles, which cover the hospital's cupola.

Levyns'kyi suffered from kyphosis. A short and smart man, he customarily called people "Sweetheart" (Ukrainian: *Serden'ko*). He once said to a worker: "Sweetheart, this wall is as humpbacked as I am."[51] He was a Ukrainian patriot and is honored as the creator (together with his employees) of the "Ukrainian Secession Style" in architecture; a philanthropist; and the founder of cultural, technical, and educational Ukrainian societies, including Prosvita (Enlightenment). His sudden death in 1919 was associated with the collapse of his enterprise during World War I and his dismissal from Lviv Technical University after the war: he refused to sign a declaration of loyalty to the reestablished Polish state.[52]

Kazimierz Julian Mokłowski

The hospital project was prepared in 1898–1901 by Levyns'kyi's Polish employee Kazimierz Julian Mokłowski (fig. 3.26). He was born in Kosów (now Kosiv) in 1869, and in 1882–1889 studied at the Secondary Technical School in Stanisławów (now Ivano-Frankivsk). In 1889, Mokłowski began his architectural studies at Lviv Technical University. As a student, he joined the Workers Party of Galicia, which was constituted as part of the Social-Democratic Workers Party of Austria in 1890 (it later became the Polish Social-Democratic Party of Galicia and Silesia). In February 1892, the university suspended him for two semesters

---

49 Ihor Zhuk, *L'viv Levyns'koho: Misto i budivnychyi* (Kyiv: Grani-T, 2010), 28–29.
50 Ibid., 79.
51 Ibid., 20.
52 Hanna Kos and Liliia Onyshchenko, *Spadshchyna velykoho budivnychoho: Profesor L'vivs'koi Politekhniky Ivan Levyns'kyi (1851–1919)* (Lviv: NU L'vivs'ka Politekhnika, 2009), passim; Zhuk, *L'viv Levyns'koho*, 51.

for engaging in "illegal assemblies and socialist propaganda."[53] Student protests and a strike followed Mokłowski's suspension, and as result he was expelled for a year. He unsuccessfully attempted to continue his studies in Vienna and Zurich and became further involved in socialist politics. He engaged in disputes with the social democrats in the circle of Rosa Luxemburg (1881–1919), who rejected the struggle for an independent Poland in favor of proletarian internationalism. Unwelcome everywhere as a radical, Mokłowski moved to Prussia and then to Saxony. His studies at the technical universities of Berlin (Charlottenburg) and Dresden were also sidelined by his political activity. In March 1894, he moved to Munich, and in August 1896, after five semesters, he graduated from the Technische Hochschule as an engineer-architect and went on to work in the city for a short time for very low wages. In 1897, because of the harsh economic conditions, Mokłowski relocated to Lviv, where Levyns'kyi employed him. He was entrusted with the Jewish Hospital project for the next three years.

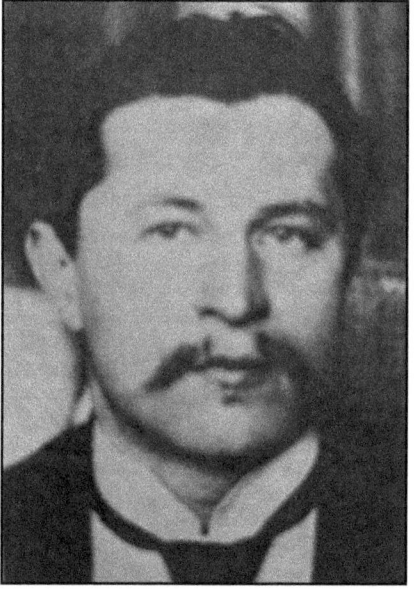

Figure 3.26. Kazimierz Mokłowski, 1869–1905. Walentyna Najdus, *Polska Partia Socjalno-demokratyczna Galicji i Śląska 1890–1919* (Warsaw: Państwowe Wydawnictwo Naukowe, 1983), 97.

In autumn 1901, before the completion of the hospital, Mokłowski became an ardent advocate of "Polish national architecture" and, in particular, the "Zakopane style" proposed by the Polish author, artist, and architect Stanisław Wyspiański (1869–1907). An

---

53 The art historian Kazimierz Mokłowski was highly valued and eagerly quoted by contemporaneous Marxist theorists. Wiesław Bieńkowski, "Mokłowski Kazimierz Julian," in *Polski Słownik Biograficzny*, vol. 21 (Warsaw: Zakład Narodowy imienia Ossolińskich, 1976), 582; Kazimierz Kelles-Krauz, "Kilka głównych zasad rozwoju sztuki," in *Poradnik dla samouków: Świat i człowiek*, vol. 5 (Warsaw: Aleksander Heflich and Stanisław Michalski, 1905), 937, 945, 948, 955, 964.

architectural theorist and Marxist thinker, Mokłowski based his ideas on Polish traditional construction and commonality of materials and techniques, rather than a highbrow architecture. He believed that the vernacular building he advocated, though only surviving in the twentieth century in the highland Podhale, was once spread throughout historic Polish lands. The traditional carpenter's knowledge, if properly studied and taught, he believed, would seed a new Polish national style and new Poland itself.

Mokłowski also called for a dramatic reassessment of architectural education; he wished to replace the "German" aesthetics of Lviv Technical University with traditional Polish carpentry, foreign intellectuals with traditional craftsmen. And he did not spare his boss: "Prof. Lewiński is an excellent practical entrepreneur, who probably has a certain sense of taste in evaluating ready-made things, but I would not insult either him or the truth by saying that he has no understanding of architecture as art."[54] In order to develop a specifically Polish architecture, Mokłowski made the radical suggestion of relocating the Department of Civil Engineering from Lviv to the more patriotic Kraków.[55]

Mokłowski's commitment to national, folk architecture—crucial, he believed, for nation states that were reemerging or coming into being for the first time—led him to studying in the field. Energetic in this work, he drafted, recorded, and photographed rural buildings in the Polish countryside. He was known for his publications, especially *Folk Art in Poland* (*Sztuka ludowa w Polsce*). He disagreed with the Jewish historian Matthias Bersohn (1824–1908), who argued that wooden synagogues in Poland were "original" Jewish designs. Mokłowski contended that there was nothing originally Jewish in such buildings and called Bersohn's claims "Jewish separatism"; he even placed the term "Jewish art" in quotation marks. He argued that the pattern for typical wooden synagogues with corner pavilions was taken from a typical Polish landlord's manor house that had disappeared in the seventeenth century and had, in its turn, been modeled on ancient wooden fortifications.[56]

No Moorish Revival work by Mokłowski is known prior to the Jewish Hospital. After his employment by Levyns'kyi, he applied his theory of national architecture to an apartment house at 38 Piekarska Street. He used bare brick and plaster to imitate the wooden logs of traditional Carpathian structures, an approach of limited circulation.

Though a man of huge stature and hearty, Mokłowski suffered from tuberculosis and, after 1900, from bone marrow inflammation. Supported by his political party, he spent the winter and spring of 1903 in Helwan, Egypt. He died in Lviv in May 1905 and was buried in Lyczakowski (Lyczakivs'kyi) Cemetery. His "pagan" (according to newspaper reports) funeral—that is, without coffin, cross, priest, or prayer—was accompanied by Polish and Ukrainian workers' choirs. One of the numerous obituaries stated: "This primordial Slav, a physical and spiritual giant, gentle, cheerful, naïve as a child, and at times mighty and

---

54 Kazimierz Mokłowski, "Dla dobra sztuki polskiej," *Krytyka* 4, no. 1 (1904): 282–283.
55 Małgorzata Kitowska-Łysiak, "Kazimierz Mokłowski (1869–1905) i jego stanowisko w sprawie tzw. stylu narodowego w architekturze Polskiej," *Lud* 70 (1986): 105–123.
56 Kazimierz Mokłowski, *Sztuka ludowa w Polsce* (Lwów: H. Altenberg, 1903), 352, 424–443; Sergey Kravtsov, "Polish-Jewish Discourse in Art History: Standpoints, Objectives, Methodologies," *Ars Judaica* (2017): 42–43.

terrible, this genius, this artist, this poet, this 'propagandist' was buried exactly as he lived and died."[57]

Judging from his life trajectory and his writings, the selection of Moorish style for the Jewish Hospital suited the client, Maurycy Lazarus, and the contractor, Ivan Levyns'kyi, rather than the architect. However, despite his personal artistic, political, and theoretical views, Mokłowski implemented this idea with great professionalism, diligence, consistency, and taste.

Michał Ulam

The next stage in the hospital's construction took place in 1911–1912 with the design and construction of the new outpatient wing (figs. 3.27 and 3.28). The commission for this freestanding building was given to the architectural firm of Michał Ulam. Michał Ulam (1879–1938, fig. 3.29) was born in Lviv to Abraham Bernard Ulam, a Jewish construction businessman whose predecessors reportedly came from Venice, and his wife Cecylia (Czajtel) née Koller. In 1901, Ulam graduated from the Industry School (Państwowa c. k. Szkoła Przemysłowa) in Lviv and studied architecture at Technische Hochschule in Munich. In 1903, after his apprenticeship with the railway engineer and architect Zygmunt Kędzierski (1839–1924) in Lviv, he established his own business.[58] Before World War I, Ulam constructed scores of educational, health care, communal, commercial, residential, transportation, and industrial buildings. He was among the first to bring the Secession (Art Nouveau) style in Lviv and "develop modern architecture, free of the deadweight of historical styles."[59] Like Levyns'kyi's company, Ulam's firm took complete responsibility for contract—from drawings, through construction and methods, to the completed building.[60]

Michał Ulam was married to Lea Leonia, daughter of the Progressive chief rabbi of Lviv, Dr. Jecheskiel Caro (1844–1915), a descendant of Joseph Caro (or Karo, 1488–1575), the author of the halakhic code *Shulḥan Arukh*.[61] In the twentieth century, the most renowned member of the family was Michał's nephew, the mathematician Stanisław Marcin Ulam (1909–1984). Stanisław Ulam belonged to the Lwów (Lviv) school of mathematics, a group of scholars renowned for their extensive contributions to point-set topology, set theory, and functional analysis. In the 1940s, when working at Los Alamos National Laboratory in New Mexico on the American hydrogen bomb, Stanisaw Ulam talked often about his uncle and Michał Ulam's addiction to gambling. These stories influenced another

---

57 M. W. K., "Listy lwowskie," *Kurjer codzienny* [Warsaw] 130 (May 25, 1905): 1.
58 "Ulam Michał," in *Almanach żydowski wydany przez Hermana Stachla, zawierający szereg artykułów wybitnych literatów, polityków i publicystów oraz życiorysy czołowych postaci Małopolski Wschodniej* (Lwów: Kultura i sztuka, 1937), 599–600; Stanislaw M. Ulam, *Adventures of a Mathematician* (Berkeley: University of California Press, 1991), 9.
59 *Budowle wykonane w dziesięcioleciu 1903-1913 przez firmę Michał Ulam architect-budowniczy, Lwów* (Lwów: Unia, 1913), unpaginated.
60 Ibid.
61 Shulḥan Arukh (in English, Set Table) is the most widely consulted legal code in Judaism. It was authored by Joseph Caro (Karo) in Safed in 1563 and published in Venice in 1565.

scientist, Nicholas Metropolis, to suggest the name for computational algorithms that rely on repeated random sampling developed by Stanisław Ulam (in collaboration with John von Neumann)—the "Monte Carlo Method."

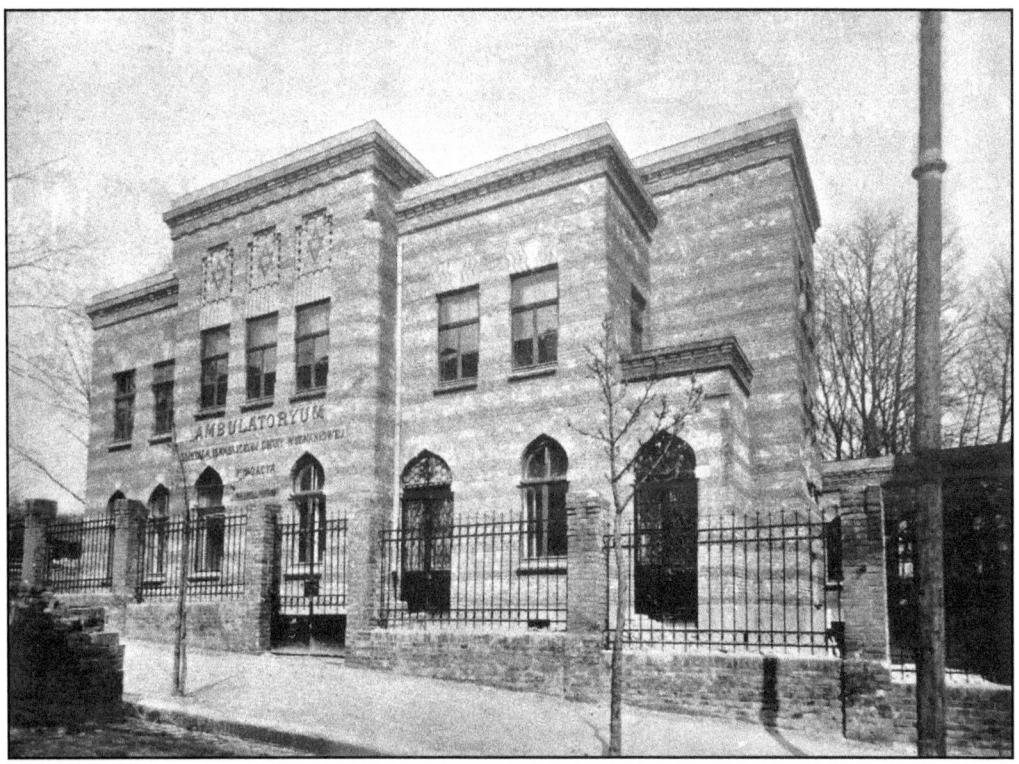

Figure 3.27. The outpatients wing of the Jewish Hospital, view from southeast. Architects Roman Feliński and Michał Ulam, 1911–1912. *Budowle wykonane w dziesięcioleciu 1903–1913 przez firmę Michał Ulam architekt-budowniczy, Lwów*, unpaginated.

Roman Feliński

The hospital's new wing was designed in 1911 by Ulam's Polish associate Roman Feliński (1886–1953, fig. 3.30). He was born in Lviv to a tailor, Feliks Feliński, and Aniela née Baurowicz. He studied at the Secondary Technical School and enrolled in the Lviv Technical University in 1903, where he passed his first state exam in 1905. He then left for studies in Munich at the Technische Hochschule, where he graduated in 1908, and completed his training in Paris in 1909. On his return home, Feliński briefly worked for Alfred Zachariewicz and Oskar Sosnowski, and in 1910–1915 for Ulam as his principal designer and supervisor. He carried out twenty-five projects in five years. He also spent eleven months abroad, developing his skills.

Ulam and Feliński were notable modernists. For instance, the Magnus department store (1912–1913) featured a concrete frame, an open plan, and modernist glazing. Their "Jewish" work in those years—such as the *beit tahara* (burial house) in the New Jewish

Cemetery (1911–1913)—was also a modernist structure. Its visual references were unrelated to any revivalism: there were only allusions to what could be considered or felt as "Jewish." In 1910, Witold Minkiewicz (1880–1961) of Lviv Technical University wrote on the emerging non-iconic approach to "native" architecture: "An assessment of what may be accepted as native belongs to the emotional sphere of the artist, which is as elusive as the very concept of the native and cannot be defined by any formula, although its existence is undeniable."[62]

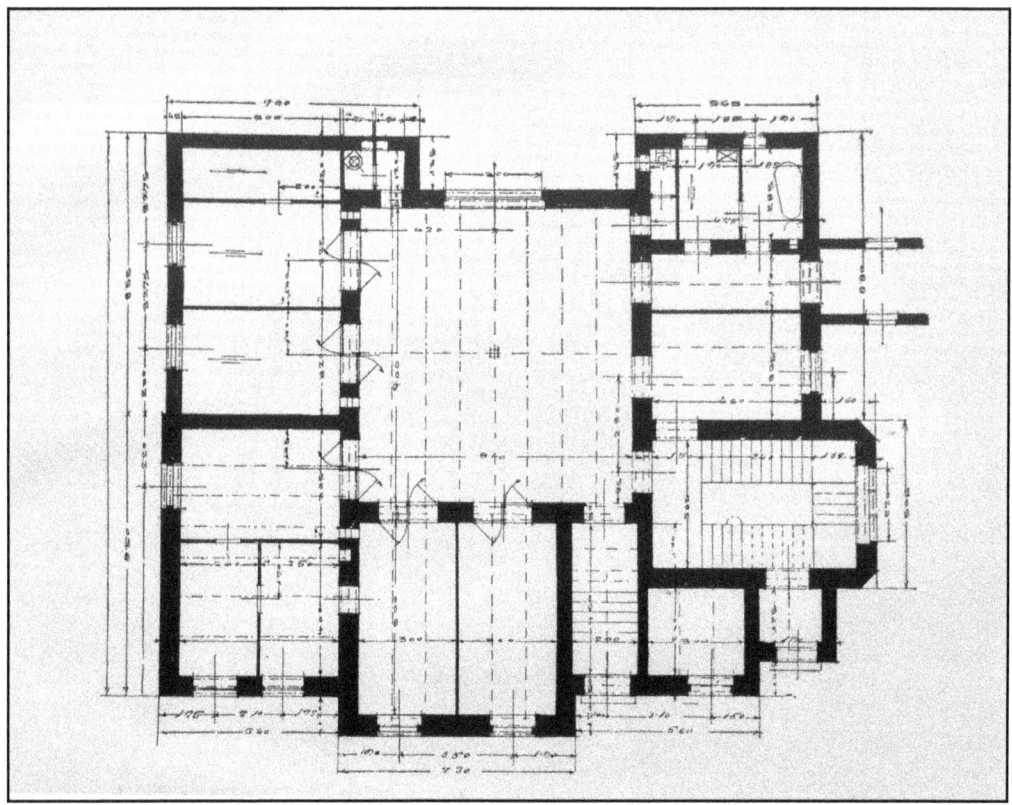

Figure 3.28. The outpatients wing of the Jewish Hospital, ground plan by architects Roman Feliński and Michał Ulam, 1911. *Budowle wykonane w dziesięcioleciu 1903–1913 przez firmę Michał Ulam architekt-budowniczy Lwów*, unpaginated.

Though modernist, Ulam's firm could take surrounding architecture into account when necessary. An example of such a project was the northern extension of St. Anna's School, the large building framing the spectacular view of the Jewish Hospital and its pointed dome from St. Anna and Kazimierzowska Streets. The new extension was seamlessly added to Hochberger's building in 1911–1913 (figs. 3.22 and 3.23). It continued the style, rhythm,

---

62 Witold Minkiewicz, "Z powodu I wystawy architektury we Lwowie," *Czasopismo techniczne* 28 (1910): 385.

fenestration, roofing, and ornamentation of its 1884 precursor without any pretension to modernism or individuality.

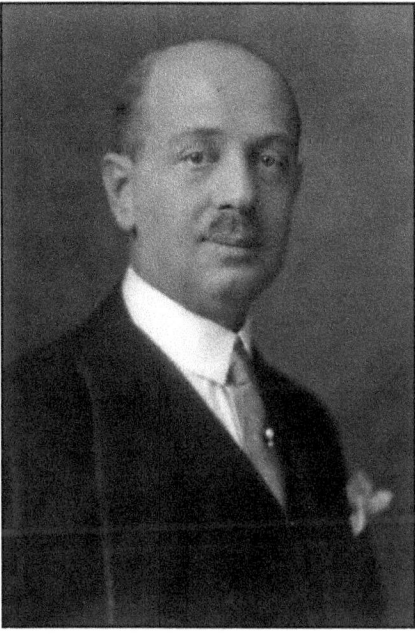

Figure 3.29. Michał Ulam, 1879–1938.[63]

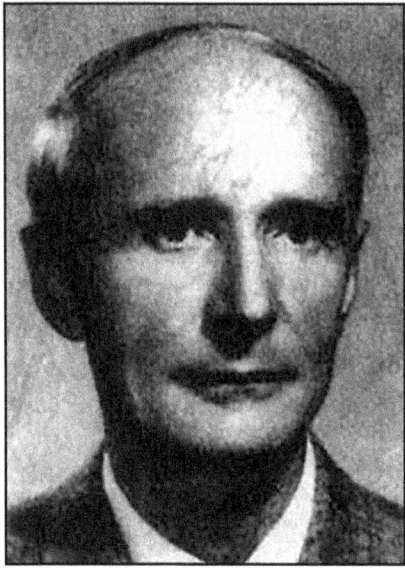

Figure 3.30. Roman Feliński, 1886–1953. Photo from ca. 1951. Archimemory. pl.

---

63 All reasonable efforts were made to locate the source of this photograph.

The new outpatient wing of the Jewish Hospital, built during the same period, was a more modernist undertaking than the extension of St. Anna's School. Located at Rappaport Street north of the main building, it featured a ground plan where symmetry was subordinate to function, dynamic massing, and concrete and steel construction. However, the overall exterior appearance was ultimately respectful towards the architectural context. The red and yellow brickwork, pointed windows, cornices, and parapet were all designed to merge the new outpatient wing with the existing Moorish Revival structure by retaining the aesthetics of the hospital proper.

***

The history of the Jewish Hospital encapsulates the development of Jewish community health care during the nineteenth and twentieth centuries. The suffering of patients was reduced, their recovery period shortened, and their stay in the hospital made more comfortable; in addition, there were improvements in hygiene and hospital staff worked with state-of-the-art equipment. And all of this was due to the generous sponsorship of Maurycy Lazarus and his wife Róża and continuous support of the wider Jewish community.

The new hospital was not simply a modern medical facility; it was a public building that both represented the Jewish community and a significant addition to the cityscape. It was constructed during the growth of nationalism throughout Europe, particularly in the Austro-Hungarian Empire—a nationalism that sought to legitimize itself through art and architecture. Though Maurycy Lazarus's political views were a long way from Jewish nationalism and Zionism, the meanings with which he imbued the Jewish Hospital were thoroughly Jewish. An example of Moorish Revival architecture, it evoked the Jewish Golden Age associated with the Romantic Historicist style of his youth.

Lazarus's team, composed of talented and European-trained Poles, Ukrainians, and Jews, reflected the ethnic composition of Lviv's artworld. Though each of the hired architects had his own ideological, business, artistic, and academic affiliations, they worked in harmony with the client's vision. Their final product took the surrounding urban landscape into careful consideration. This situational awareness, and longing for propriety and continuity, was highly appreciated in fin de siècle Lviv. While conservative rather than revolutionary, Lviv's aesthetic preferences went hand in hand with a commitment to social and technical progress. It was this restrained progressiveness which shaped the growing city, its institutions, and buildings.

Archival Sources

TsDIAL
Fond 701, op. 2, spr. 1559, f. 55.

Bibliography

Bałaban, Majer. "Szpital żydowski we Lwowie." *Wschód* 108 (1902): 3–5.

Bieńkowski, Wiesław. "Mokłowski Kazimierz Julian." In *Polski Słownik Biograficzny*, vol. 21, 582–585. Warsaw: Zakład Narodowy imienia Ossolińskich & Wydawnictwo Polskiej Akademii Nauk, 1976.

Biriulow, Jurij [Biryulov, Yuri]. *Lwów: Ilustrowany przewodnik*. Lviv: Centrum Europy, 2003.

_____. *Rzeźba lwowska od połowy XVIII wieku do 1939 roku*. Warsaw: Neriton, 2007.

_____. *Yevreis'ka arkhitekturna spadshchyna L'vova*. Lviv: Vydavnytstvo Staroho Leva, 2022.

Budowle wykonane w dziesięcioleciu 1903-1913 przez firmę Michał Ulam architekt-budowniczy, Lwów. Lwów: Unia, 1913.

Chipiez, Charles, and Georges Perrot. *Le Temple de Jérusalem et la Maison du Bois-Liban restitués d'après Ezéchiel et le Livre des Rois*. Paris: Hachette, 1889.

Feuerstein, Henryk. "Lazarus, życie i czyny lwowskiego filantropa." In *Almanach żydowski wydany przez Hermana Stachla, zawierający szereg artykułów wybitnych literatów, polityków i publicystów oraz życiorysy czołowych postaci Małopolski Wschodniej*, 216–219. Lwów: Kultura i sztuka, 1937.

[Förster, Ludwig]. "Die Baron Pereira'sche Willa aus der Herrschaft Königstetten im Tullnerboden nächst Wien." *Allgemeine Bauzeitung* (1849): 107.

_____. "Das israelitische Bethhaus in der Wiener Vorstadt Leopoldstadt." *Allgemeine Bauzeitung* (1859): 14–16.

Glembotskaya, Galina. *Khudozhniki-evrei L'vova pervoi poloviny XX veka: Zhizn', tvorchestvo, sud'ba*. Lviv: Stavropigion, 2015.

Kalmar, Ivan D. "Orientalism, the Jews, and Synagogue Architecture." *Jewish Social Studies*, n.s., 7, no. 3 (Spring–Summer, 2001): 68–100.

Kapral, Miron [ed]. *Privilegia Civitatis Leopoliensis (XIV–XVIII Saec.)*. Lviv: Dokumental'na skarbnytsia L'vova, 1998.

Kelles-Krauz, Kazimierz. "Kilka głównych zasad rozwoju sztuki." In *Poradnik dla samouków: Świat i człowiek*, 887–1013. Warsaw: Aleksander Heflich and Stanisław Michalski, 1905.

Kitowska-Łysiak, Małgorzata. "Kazimierz Mokłowski (1869–1905) i jego stanowisko w sprawie tzw. stylu narodowego w architekturze polskiej." *Lud* 70 (1986): 105–123.

Klimashevs'kyi, Andrii, ed. *Keramichnyi kod Ivana Levyns'koho v estetychnomu vymiri ukraintsia XIX – pochatku XX st*. Lviv: Rarytety Ukrainy, 2020.

Kos, Hanna, and Liliia Onyshchenko. *Spadshchyna velykoho budivnychoho: Profesor L'vivs'koi Politekhniky Ivan Levyns'kyi (1851–1919)*. Lviv: L'vivs'ka Politekhnika, 2009.

Kravtsov, Sergey R. "Jewish Identities in Synagogue Architecture of Galicia and Bukovina." *Ars Judaica: The Bar-Ilan Journal of Jewish Art* 6 (2010): 81–100.

_____. "Polish-Jewish Discourse in Art History: Standpoints, Objectives, Methodologies." *Ars Judaica: The Bar-Ilan Journal of Jewish Art* 13 (2017): 39–48.

"Kronika." *Kurjer lwowski* 269 (October 25, 1902): 3–4.

Łoza, Stanisław. *Słownik architektów i budowniczych Polaków oraz cudzoziemców w Polsce pracujących*. Warsaw: Kasa im. Mianowskiego Instytutu Popierania Nauki, 1931.

M. W. K. "Listy lwowskie." *Kurjer codzienny* [Warsaw] 130 (May 25, 1905): 1.

Mehrer, Henryk. *Szpital lwowskiej gminy wyznaniowej izraelickiej fundacyi Maurycego Lazarusa*. Lwów: Szpital Lwowskiej Gminy Wyzn. Izraelickiej, 1906.

Mokłowski, Kazimierz. "Dla dobra sztuki polskiej." *Krytyka* 4, no. 1 (1904): 279–284.

———. *Sztuka ludowa w Polsce*. Lwów: H. Altenberg, 1903.

Muthesius, Stefan. "Renate Wagner-Rieger and Mara Reissenberg, *Theophil von Hansen* (Die Wiener Ringstrasse, Bild einer Epoche, vol. 4, Section VIII) (Wiesbaden, 1980)." *The Journal of the Society of Architectural Historians* 42, no. 1 (1983): 80–81

Piotrowski, Josef. *Lemberg und Umgebung (Żółkiew, Podhorce, Brzeżany und and.). Handbuch für Kunstliebhaber und Reisende*. Lwów: H. Altenberg, G. Seyfarth, E. Wende & Co, 1916.

Prokopovych, Markian. *Habsburg Lemberg: Architecture, Public Space, and Politics in the Galician Capital, 1772–1914*. West Lafayette: Purdue University Press, 2009.

Sas-Zubrzycki, Jan. *Zabytki miasta Lwowa*. Lwów: Nakładem autora, 1928.

Schorsch, Ismar. "The Myth of Sephardic Supremacy." *Leo Baeck Institute Year Book* 34, no. 1 (January 1989): 47–66.

Simferovska, Anastasiia. "L'vivs'kyi portret pershoi polovyny XX stolittia: Khudozhnia representatsiia osobystosti." Ph.D. diss., L'vivs'ka Natsional'na Akademiia Mystetstv, 2018.

"Sprawozdanie ze zgromadzenia odb. d. 29 stycznia r.b." *Czasopismo techniczne* 14, no. 5 (1896): 57–58.

"Szpital izraelicki fundacji Maurycego Lazarusa." *Gazeta Lwowska* 130 (June 9, 1903): 4.

"Ulam Michał." In *Almanach żydowski wydany przez Hermana Stachla, zawierający szereg artykułów wybitnych literatów, polityków i publicystów oraz życiorysy czołowych postaci Małopolski Wschodniej*, 599–600. Lwów: Kultura i sztuka, 1937.

Ulam, Stanislaw M. *Adventures of a Mathematician*. Berkeley: University of California Press, 1991.

Vuitsyk, Volodymyr. "Narodnyi Dim u L'vovi." In *Visnyk instytutu "Ukrzakhidproektrestavratsiia,"* 14:164–165. Lviv: Ukrzakhidproektrestavratsiia, 2004.

Wiczkowski, Józef. *Lwów, jego rozwój i stan kulturalny oraz przewodnik po mieście*. Lwów: Wydział gospodarczy X. zjazdu lekarzy i przyrodników polskich, oraz reprezentacji m. Lwowa, 1907.

Zhuk, Ihor. *L'viv Levyns'koho: Misto i budivnychyi*. Kyiv: Grani-T, 2010.

Zimorowicz, Bartołomiej. *Potriynyi L'viv: Leopolis Triplex*, Ukrainian trans. Natalia Tsariova. Lviv: Tsentr Evropy, 2002.

Chapter 4

The Maurycy Lazarus Foundation Israelite Hospital (1903–1939)

Anna Jakimyszyn-Gadocha

At the turn of the nineteenth century, prominent European physicians began efforts to improve hygiene among the urban population. The constant progress of knowledge and, in particular, the development of the medical sciences, lead to attempts to control epidemic infectious diseases. This coincided with government policies, dating back to the early nineteenth century, aimed at implementing measures to improve the health and life of the population.[1] These changes also affected Lviv—an important center of political, scientific, cultural, social, and economic activity, a multicultural and multireligious city—which from 1772 (the First Partition of Poland) until World War I remained under Habsburg rule.

Health-oriented policies in Lviv (1867–1914)

Lviv already had waterworks in the fifteenth century, brick wells, sewers, and cobblestones. In the seventeenth century there were three hospitals in the city. Unfortunately, from the mid-seventeenth century, due to constant external threats and numerous wars, this infrastructure was not properly maintained and developed. After the First Partition of Poland, no investments were made that could have improved the city's dire sanitary conditions. Only the regulation of the riverbed of the Poltva (Pełtew) in its upper reaches improved sanitation. The construction of several canals prevented sewage from seeping into the groundwater. Water was brought in through the Węgliński and Mariacki waterworks, and

---

1   Krzysztof Broński, "Galicja w dobie autonomii wobec wyzwań nowoczesności," in *Między zacofaniem a modernizacją. Społeczno-gospodarcze problemy ziem polskich na przestrzeni wieków*, ed. Elżbieta Kościk and Tomasz Głowiński (Wrocław: Gajt Wydawnictwo, 2009), 395–412.

in place of the parish cemeteries, a large municipal cemetery was created in Lychakiv. Major changes, however, began to be made during the period of Galician autonomy (1867–1914).[2]

During that time, the public health care was overseen by the central authorities in Vienna and the autonomous authorities in Lviv. Vienna was involved in the establishment of the legal and organizational foundations of public health care structure and in active efforts to ensure the smooth functioning of the structures thus established. Lviv's local government was responsible for sanitation (garbage removal, etc.), epidemiological prevention, and health care in the city. In 1872, a municipal health department was established. The city was divided into health districts. Doctors assigned to the districts provided free medical assistance, looked after those suffering from infectious diseases, and performed autopsies. In 1893, the Lviv Rescue Society was founded to intervene in cases of sudden illness and accidents.[3]

From the 1870s onwards, tuberculosis and infectious diseases (particularly smallpox, diphtheria, and typhoid fever) caused the greatest number of deaths in the city.[4] In order to reduce morbidity and mortality, as well as improve sanitary conditions, measures were taken to combat infectious diseases, and recommendations were made about the cleanliness of buildings and the environment. New streets were laid out, making sure they were wide and paved with stone or wooden cubes. Sidewalks were covered with stone slabs, and roadside ditches were eliminated. Municipal services responsible for street cleaning were organized. Parks, squares, and playgrounds were created. Beginning in the 1880s, a vaccination campaign began, primarily against smallpox. The food hygiene (including places where food was sold) was supervised (since 1881 the town had employed a chemist to test food and water). A municipal slaughterhouse was opened in 1901, and the Municipal Maintenance Service was established in 1909. There was also a successful development of the town's sewage system and water supply. Access to medical care was expanded and, gradually, the number of practicing physicians in the city increased. In 1870 there were about fifty; by the end of 1895 there were 168 physicians and eighteen masters of surgery.[5]

As a result, from 1890 to 1910 the annual mortality rate in Lviv decreased. In 1890 there were thirty deaths per one thousand inhabitants, while in 1910 there were twenty-one

---

2 Julian Dybiec, "Galicja na drodze do wielkiej przemiany," in *Kraków i Galicja wobec przemian cywilizacyjnych (1866–1914). Studia i szkice*, ed. Krzysztof Fiołek and Marian Stala (Kraków: Towarzystwo Autorów i Wydawców Prac Naukowych Universitas 2011), 31–42; Julian Dybiec, "Nauka a modernizacja społeczna w Galicji w epoce autonomii," in *Galicja i jej dziedzictwo*, vol. 20, *Historia wychowania, misja i edukacja*, ed. Kazimierz Szmyd and Julian Dybiec (Rzeszów: Wydawnictwo Uniwersytetu Rzeszowskiego 2008), 58–65.
3 Łukasz T. Sroka, *Rada Miejska we Lwowie w okresie autonomii galicyjskiej 1870–1914. Studium o elicie władzy* (Kraków: Wydawnictwo Naukowe Uniwersytetu Pedagogicznego, 2012), 177.
4 Konrad Wnęk, "Przemiany demograficzne we Lwowie w latach 1829–1938," *Zeszyty Naukowe Uniwersytetu Jagiellońskiego. Prace Historyczne* 135 (2008): 116–117.
5 Antoni Pawlikowski, "Stosunki zdrowotne," in *Miasto Lwów w okresie samorządu 1870–1895*, ed. Edmund Mochnacki (Lwów: Z drukarni W. A. Szyjkowskiego nakł. Gminy Król. Stoł. Miasta Lwowa, 1896), 269–271. Sroka, *Rada Miejska we Lwowie*, 180–185.

deaths per one thousand inhabitants.[6] However, the rate was still high; in 1910 in Vienna, for example, there were 16.8 deaths per one thousand.[7]

General and private hospitals in Galicia

In December 1869, during the period of Galician autonomy, the operation of public hospitals was regulated by the Galician Sejm (National Galician Parliament); and the municipal law was passed in February 1891. The regulations mainly concerned rules for financing hospitals and the manner in which they were managed, especially by so-called hospital councils. On January 6, 1875, the Galician Parliament passed a law on the free treatment for the poor. On July 6, 1897, a national law was passed defining rules for general and public hospitals, as well as maternity institutions and establishments for the mentally ill (called insane persons, at the time). The activities of the Galician health service were also determined by other lower-ranking regulations (ordinances and circulars, e.g., on not admitting terminally ill people to the hospitals—dated 1869, 1880, 1882) and service instructions for individual hospitals issued by the National Department of Galicia.

In addition to general hospitals, there were also private hospitals in Galicia, and their number exceeded the former. These included private facilities (owned, for example, by doctors), facilities financed by local (county and municipal) authorities, religious hospitals, hospitals run by industrial enterprises, and hospitals founded by various foundations. In 1873, there were thirty-four private hospitals in Galicia; by 1896, there were already fifty-four, located in forty-five towns and cities. Twelve of them were in the hands of Jewish communities. These were hospitals in Brody, Yaroslav, Kolomyia, Kraków, Lviv, Przemyśl, Rzeszów, Sambor, Ternopil, Tarnów, Zalishchyky, Zbarazh, and Zolochiv.[8]

Hospitals in Lviv

In 1895, Lviv had hospitals run by the state, the city, and privately; there were also eight clinics. To these should be added additional five city charitable institutions for: cripples (according to the terminology of the time), poor Christians, and orphans. There was also a hospice for men, another for women, and five orphanages. In addition, there were fourteen private establishments for orphans, the disabled, the poor, and the elderly.[9] However, it

---

6 See: Konrad Wnęk and Lidia A. Zyblikiewicz and Ewa Callahan, *Ludność nowoczesnego Lwowa w latach 1857–1938* (Kraków: Tow. Nauk. Societas Vistulana 2006).
7 Sroka, *Rada Miejska we Lwowie*, 177–185.
8 Piotr Franaszek, *Zdrowie publiczne w Galicji w dobie autonomii (Wybrane problemy)* (Kraków: Wydawnictwo Uniwersytetu Jagiellońskiego 2002), 152.
9 Pawlikowski, "Stosunki zdrowotne," 275–276.

should be noted that the hospitals of the time treated almost exclusively poor people who could not afford individual medical care (for additional details, see table on page 37).

Three Lviv hospitals were given the status of public and general hospitals. These were: the National General Hospital, also known as the Main Hospital, the Institution for the Mentally Ill in Kulparkov, and St. Sophia Children's Hospital. The first of the aforementioned hospitals was the largest medical hospital in the city.[10] It was not available to Jews until the 1870s, when a 1829s prohibition on admitting Jews was lifted. The Galician Parliament considered the prohibition contrary to state laws regarding the equality of all residents of the Austro-Hungarian Empire and, in particular, the right to admit patients to state hospitals.[11] Opened on June 7, 1903, the Maurycy Lazarus Foundation Israelite Hospital (fig. 4.1), known as Lazarus Hospital or the Jewish Hospital, was classified as a private and religious hospital.[12]

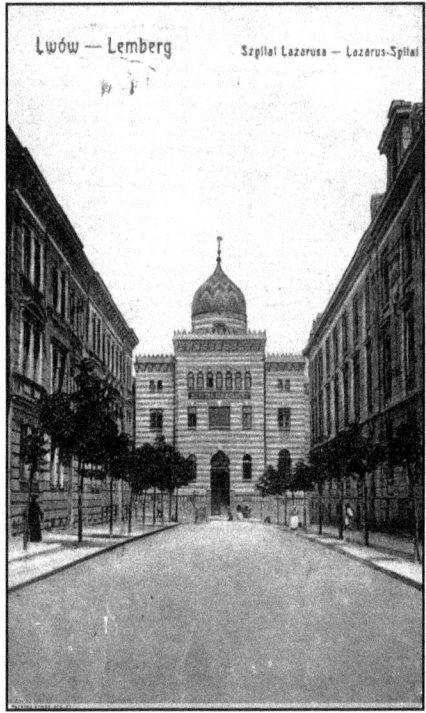

Figure 4.1. The Maurycy Lazarus Foundation Israelite Hospital. ÖNB, Bildarchiv und Grafiksammlung, AK001_508.

---

10 In 1885, there were 638 beds in all departments of the hospital; five years later, there were 650 beds; in 1891, there were 700; and in 1896, there were 835; Piotr Franaszek, "Krajowy szpital powszechny we Lwowie na przełomie XIX i XX wieku," *Zeszyty Naukowe Uniwersytetu Jagiellońskiego. Prace Historyczne* 127 (2000): 129.
11 Ibid.: 127.
12 For more about Jewish patrons in Lviv: Łukasz T. Sroka, "Zaangażowanie społeczne elit żydowskich we Lwowie w okresie autonomii galicyjskiej," in *L'viv: Misto – suspil'stvo – kul'tura*, vol. 8, Chastyna 1: *Vlada i suspil'stvo*, ed. Olena Arkusha and Marian Mudryi, *Visnyk L'vivs'koho universytetu. Seriya istorychna* (Lviv: L'vivs'kyi Derzhavnyi Universytet imeni Ivana Franka, 2012), 351–364.

Not only a Jewish hospital . . .

The year 1903 was significant in the history of Lviv's hospitals not only because of the establishment of a Jewish institution, but also because of the initiative of Archbishop Andrey Sheptytsky (1865–1944), (fig. 4.2) a Greek Catholic clergyman who served as archbishop metropolitan of Lviv and Halych in 1900–1944. In a one-story building located at the foot of St. George's Hill, Sheptytsky opened a free clinic; it was for all the sick of Lviv and Galicia. This was the first such Greek Catholic enterprise in Galicia.

The institution grew in the interwar period, moving to a building on Piotr Skarga Street build for its needs. It was named the Metropolitan Andrey Sheptytsky Hospital "Narodna Lichnytsya," thus commemorating its founder.[13]

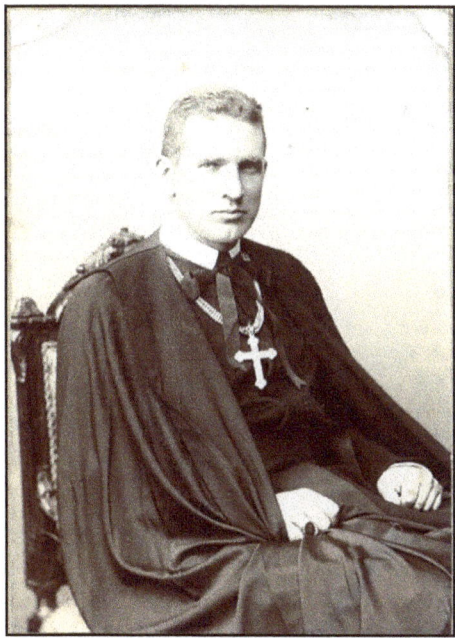

Figure 4.2. Andrey Sheptytsky, 1901. Photo: E. Trzemeski.

Three cities, three modern Jewish hospitals

Maurycy Lazarus aimed to create a modern hospital. For this reason, during his travels in Europe, he familiarized himself with the principles of other medical institutions. This was all the more important because the nineteenth century saw changes in the way hospitals were designed and operated.

---

13 Oleksandr Kitsera, "Mytropolyt Andrey Sheptyts'kyy i 'Narodna lichnytsya,'" *Likars'kyy zbirnyk. Nova seriya* 13 (2004): 66–74. Nataliya Matlashenko, "Narodna lichnytsya – persha ukrayinska likarnya v Halychyni," *Farmatsevt praktyk* (2015), http://fp.com.ua/articles/ narodna-lichnitsya-persha-ukrayinska-likarnya-v-galichini.

Since the second half of the eighteenth century, physicians had demonstrated the close relationship between the mortality rate and sanitary conditions existing in medical institutions.[14] In the nineteenth century, modern hospitals were built on the plan of an elongated rectangle. The central part of the building on the ground floor housed administrative and outpatient functions. The first floor contained state-of-the-art operating rooms. The wings of the building contained small patient rooms, bathrooms, and toilets. The rooms were well lit, well ventilated, and heated.[15] New Jewish hospitals were similar.

The first modern Jewish hospital was built in Kraków. Its construction was initiated by Dr. Józef Oettinger (see chapter 1) a graduate of the Faculty of Medicine at Jagiellonian University, head of the Jewish hospital operating in Kraków since the 1820s, and later an associate professor of the history of medicine at Jagiellonian University.[16] (fig. 4.3)

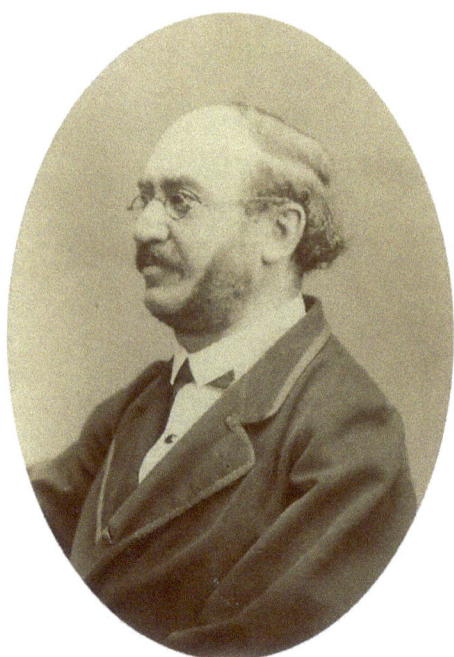

Figure 4.3. Portrait of Józef Oettinger. Atelier of W. Rzewuski. PAU, Legacy of J. Majer, RKPS.6624 k.52.

Financial considerations stood in the way of the project's completion. As the Jewish community did not have adequate funds, it borrowed money from Emperor Franz Joseph I,

---

14 Robert Frédéric Bridgman, *L'hôpital et la Cité* (Paris: Editions du Cosmos, 1963).
15 Elżbieta Waszczyszyn, "The Changes in 19th Century European Hospital Architecture. Selected Examples," *Technical Transactions Architecture* 3-A (2015): 180–181.
16 Jerzy Strojnowski, "Józef Oettinger, pierwszy habilitowany docent i profesor historii medycyny na polskim uniwersytecie," *Kwartalnik Historii Nauki i Techniki* 15 (1970): 57–69.

among others. Jewish and non-Jewish individuals also donated to the project.[17] The old hospital had eighteen beds, and forty by the 1840s.[18] The new facility, designed by architect Antoni Stacherski, was to have one hundred beds.[19] Work began in the garden of the existing hospital in 1861 and was completed between 1866 and 1876.[20] (fig. 4.4). In 1881, the hospital had fifty beds for internal diseases only. In 1897, surgical, psychiatric, and children's departments were opened. The year 1899 was marked by the opening of a department for women's diseases and the installation of a chemical and bacteriological laboratory.[21]

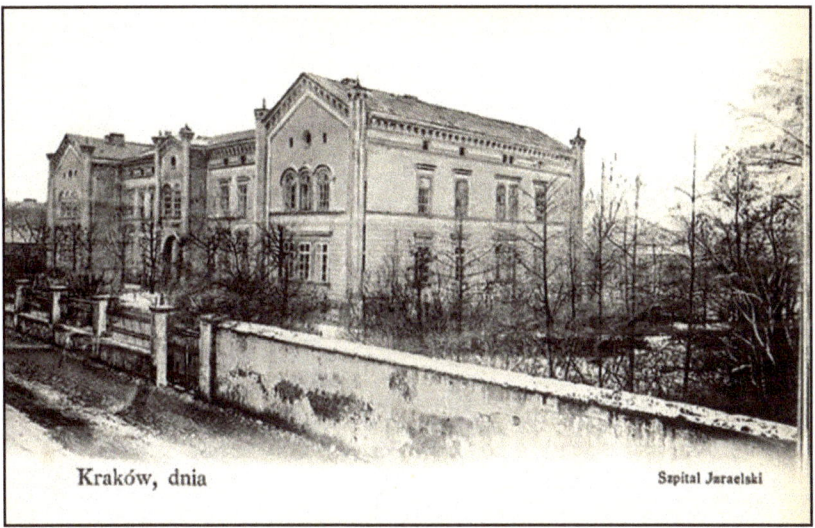

Figure 4.4. Jewish Hospital in Kraków (nineteenth century). ANK, Collection of postcards, C-V-23.

The second modern Jewish hospital was established in Vienna. It was to replace, with forty beds, the hospital founded by Samuel Oppeheimer in 1698.[22] It was built on the newly delineated Währinger Gürtelstraße (today: Währinger Gürtel). The building, whose construction was financed by Baron Anselm Salomon von Rothschild (1803–1874),[23] was to commemorate his father Salomon Freiherr von Rothschild (1774–1855), the businessman, banker, and progenitor of the Austrian branch of the Rothschild family.

---

17 Aleksander B. Skotnicki, *Szpital Gminy Wyznaniowej Żydowskiej w Krakowie 1866–1941* (Kraków: Stradomskie Centrum Dialogu, 2013), 7.
18 Anna Jakimyszyn, *Żydzi krakowscy w dobie Rzeczypospolitej Krakowskiej: status prawny, przeobrażenia gminy, system edukacyjny* (Kraków: Wydawnictwo Austeria, 2008), 174, 179.
19 ANK, sign. ABM 42, district VIII, 1, f. 37.
20 Barbara Zbroja, *Miasto umarłych: architektura publiczna Żydowskiej Gminy Wyznaniowej w Krakowie w latach 1868–1939* (Kraków: Wydawnictwo WAM, 2005), 39–40.
21 Skotnicki, *Szpital Gminy*, 8–9.
22 Bernhard Wölfler, *Das alte und neue Wiener Israeliten-Spital nach authentischen Quellen dargestellt* (Wien: Gerold, 1873), 2.
23 Ibid., 2.

Called the Rothschild-Spital or Spital der israelitischen Kultusgemeinde in Wien, the hospital was designed by the Jewish architect Wilhelm Stiassny (1842–1910; see chapter three). It opened in 1873,[24] and had one hundred beds. At the time, it was the most modern hospital in the city, as it was built according to the latest advances in hospital design. Representatives of the religious community, doctors, and the director of the old hospital had visited sixty-one hospitals in nineteen cities across Europe and communicated their findings to Stiassny. In 1903, a surgical and gynecological wing with fifty beds and an outpatient clinic was opened at Rothschild-Spital. New outpatient departments soon followed: ophthalmology (1906), a clinic for "the nervously ill" (1907), dermatology (1912), and laryngology clinic. From 1908, the Empress Elisabeth Institute for Israelite Nurses, where Jewish women and girls were trained as nurses, was also based at the hospital.[25]

The Jewish Hospital in Lviv was the third modern medical facility owned by the Jewish community, and the second, after Kraków, to be located in Galicia.[26] The possibility of acquiring medical education in Vienna, Kraków, and Lviv, and family and professional contacts between members of the aforementioned Jewish communities made Vienna, Kraków, and Lviv hospitals leading centers for the training of new medical staff and the implementation of modern research methods.[27]

The Lazarus Jewish Hospital before World War I

The rules of the hospital were set forth in the founding document of 1899.[28] There were also internal regulations, which covered all matters concerning the hospital's operations. The hospital also had extensive auxiliary facilities: kitchen, pantries, a mangle, a linen and clothing store for patients, rooms for disinfecting hospital equipment, and a dissecting room. The hospital buildings also housed rooms for employees (primarily auxiliary and technical staff).[29]

The director of the Jewish Hospital was always a physician; he would supervise the medical and nursing staff, as well as the administrative and custodial personnel. He sat on the Hospital Council. The hospital management dealt with administration and billing, undertook all the clerical tasks necessary for admitting patients, and maintained patient medical records. Furthermore, it handled correspondence, supplies for the kitchen, storerooms,

---

24 The hospital operated according to the rules established in 1871. See: *Organisations-Statut fuer das Spital der Israelitischen Kultusgemeinde in Wien* (Wien: Selbstverlage der Direction 1871).
25 Michael Heindl and Ruth Koblizek, *125 Jahre Rothschild-Spital* (Wien: Dagobert Wien, 1998).
26 Jacek Purchla, "Kraków i Lwów: zmienność relacji w XIX i XX wieku," in *Kraków i Lwów w cywilizacji europejskiej: materiały międzynarodowej konferencji zorganizowanej w dniach 15–16 listopada 2002*, ed. Jacek Purchla and Marta Dyhas (Kraków: Międzynarodowe Centrum Kultury, 2003), 81–90.
27 See: Łukasz T. Sroka, *In the light of Vienna: Jews in Lviv—Between Tradition and Modernisation (1867–1914)* (Berlin: Peter Lang, 2018).
28 TsDIAL, fond 701, op. 2, spr. 1559, f. 50–59.
29 Anna Jakimyszyn-Gadocha, *W trosce o zdrowie żydowskiej społeczności Lwowa (1918–1939)* (Kraków: Wydawnictwo Austeria, 2021), 57.

and laundry, and oversaw the hospital's general cleanliness. The hospital's finances were overseen by the Hospital Council, which consisted of subcommittees that supervised the nursing home, the cemetery's financial affairs, funerals, ritual baths, and real estate. Its members were appointed by the Jewish Community Council.[30]

The medical staff was small. Four doctors worked in two departments (internal medicine and surgery, comprising one hundred beds) and six doctors worked in the outpatient clinics.[31] There is no data on the number of nursing staff. The four internal medicine and surgery doctors—Henryk Mehrer (fig. 4.5) Salomon Ruff (fig. 4.6) David Ehrlich (fig. 4.7), and Wilhelm Pisek (fig. 4.8)—were in contact with each other not only at the Jewish Hospital, where they worked together for decades to come, but also at other medical institutions operating in the city. They were also united by their activities in Jewish and non-Jewish professional (medical), charitable, and welfare associations.

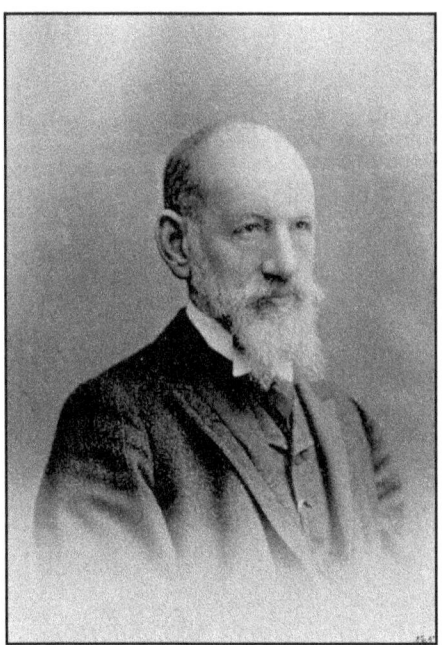

Figure 4.5. Dr. Henryk Mehrer. Henryk Mehrer, *Szpital lwowskiej gminy wyznaniowej izraelickiej fundacyi Maurycego Lazarusa* (Lwów: Szpital Lwowskiej Gminy Wyzn. Izraelickiej, 1906), 34.

Dr. Mehrer and Dr. Ruff worked in the internal medicine department. Dr. Mehrer[32] began at the Jewish Hospital in the 1880s. Initially, he was a deputy chief surgeon, but

---

30 Ibid., 62, 443–444.
31 Henryk Feuerstein, "Trzydzieści lat szpitala fundacji błp. Maurycego Lazarusa (Reportaż ze wspomnień, cyfr i faktów)," in *Almanach zdrowia TOZ-u i Szpitala Żydowskiego fundacji Maurycego Lazarusa* (Lwów: TOZ, 1937), 12; Henryk Mehrer, *Szpital lwowskiej gminy wyznaniowej izraelickiej fundacyi Maurycego Lazarusa* (Lwów: Szpital Lwowskiej Gminy Wyzn. Izraelickiej, 1906), 12.
32 At different stages of his life, Dr. Mehrer used different variants of his first name: Herschl, Heinrich, Henry. He was a native of Lviv (born in 1846) and was educated in Vienna, where he graduated in the early 1870s. Mehrer, *Szpital lwowskiej gminy*, 40.

in time took over as head of the surgical department.³³ In 1903, he assumed the duties of director of the hospital and served as both its director and head of internal medicine. He was the author of a brochure on the history and activities of the hospital, which was published in Lviv in 1906.³⁴ Dr. Salomon (Stanislaw) Ruff (1872–1941) worked in the surgical clinic at Lviv University under Dr. Ludwik Rydygier (until 1904), then became head of the surgical department of the Jewish Hospital, and also had duties in the surgical department at Lviv General Polyclinic. For many years he was active in the Lviv Medical Society, serving as its vice president (twice) and president (from 1932). He was decorated for his activities, in 1928 receiving the Officer's Cross of the Order of Polonia Restituta, the second-highest civilian decoration awarded by the Polish authorities for outstanding achievement in education, science, sports, culture, art, economy, defense of the country, social activities, state service, and the development of good relations with other countries. In July 1941, Ruff was murdered by Nazi German occupation forces with a group of scholars on the Wuleckie Hills.³⁵

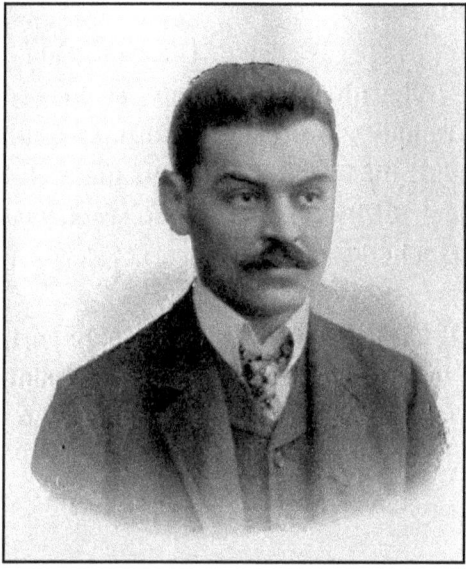

Figure 4.6. Dr Salomon Ruff. Mehrer, *Szpital lwowskiej gminy*, 35.

Dr. Dawid Ehrlich and Dr. Wilhelm Pisek worked in the internal medicine department. Dr. Ehrlich (1866 Lviv–1939?) was an internist and diagnostician. He was educated in his hometown and in Vienna (he received his diploma in 1899). Professionally, he was

---

33 Ibid.
34 Ibid.
35 *Almanach żydowski wydany przez Hermana Stachla zawierający szereg artykułów wybitnych literatów, polityków i publicystów oraz życiorysy czołowych postaci Małopolski Wschodniej* (Lwów: Wydawnictwo Kultura i Sztuka, 1937), 422–423. Teresa Ostrowska, "Stanisław Ruff," in *Polski Słownik Biograficzny* (Wrocław: Zakład Narodowy im. Ossolińskich - Wydawnictwo Polskiej Akademii Nauk, 1991), 65.

associated not only with the Jewish Hospital, where he served as the head of the internal medicine department, but also with the National General Hospital (1889–1891).[36] His wartime fate remains unknown—the last reference to him is from 1939.[37] His colleague from the department, Dr. Wilhelm Pisek (1856 Kraków–1939), received his medical diploma in Kraków (1878), worked at the National General Hospital in Lviv, and was head of the Internal Medicine Department at Lviv Polyclinic. During World War I, he headed the Red Cross hospital in Lviv, and later, in Vienna, he ran the internal ward of a military hospital. He was a member of the Lviv City Council. For many years, he served as president of the Lviv Medical Society. He was also a member of the Society of Czech Physicians and the author of more than thirty scientific papers.[38] He died in Lviv on July 22, 1939.[39]

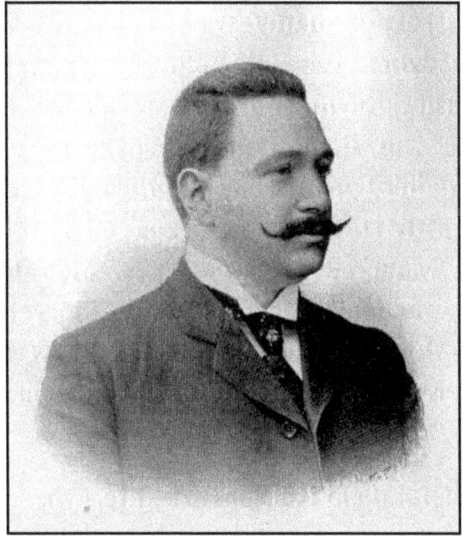

Figure 4.7. Dr. Dawid Ehrlich. Mehrer, *Szpital lwowskiej gminy*, 39.

The medical staff cared for a large number of patients, who had to comply with regulations concerning behavior on hospital premises (for example, there was a total ban on smoking). The hospital divided patients according to their financial status: those who were poor and lived in the Lviv municipality were guaranteed free treatment in the hospital, while others were charged a fee for their rooms and medical services received. All patients had to agree to rules regarding conduct during visits and admissions. Moreover, during a stay in the hospital, a patient could use only hospital equipment and all personal belongings were

---

36 *Almanach żydowski*, 380–381.
37 Józef Krętowski, *Ich pamięci . . . Straty osobowe lekarzy na Kresach Rzeczypospolitej w latach drugiej wojny światowej* (Białystok: Skryba, 2018), 63.
38 *Almanach żydowski*, 418–420.
39 Krętowski, *Ich pamięci*, 143.

deposited in the hospital office. All furnishings in patient and staff rooms (cabinets, stools, metal beds, etc.) were lacquered white to maintain cleanliness and sterile conditions.

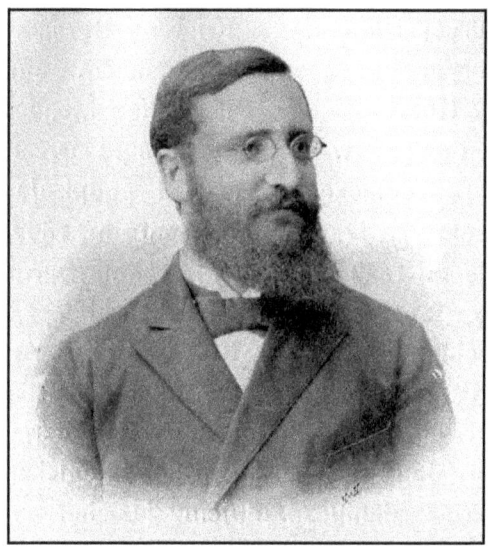

Figure 4.8. Wilhelm Pisek. Mehrer, *Szpital lwowskiej gminy*, 38.

Proper nutrition was an important part of treatment and recovery. As a result, meals were high in calories and contained plenty of protein, carbohydrates and seasonal fruits and vegetables. They were prepared in the hospital kitchen, served at fixed times (five times a day), and delivered to patient rooms via dumbwaiters.

For many in the Jewish community, especially Orthodox Jews, the hospital represented an opportunity to preserve their traditions and beliefs. Indeed, hospital patients were guaranteed kosher meals. (Even though there was a charitable association in Lviv dedicated to providing kosher food to those in hospitals, its activities were limited). Equally important for many patients was the hospital's synagogue (fig. 4.9). For this reason, Jews belonging to the Lviv religious community, as well as those from further afield, favored the Jewish Hospital. From the 1870s onward, there was a steady increase in the number of Jewish residents in Lviv: in 1900 there were 44,254 (27 percent of the city's total population); ten years later, there were 57,387 (29 percent of Lviv's total population).[40] Even when the Jewish Hospital opened, it did not have enough beds to serve the Jewish population of the city. Non-Jews also benefited from the medical assistance there. In fact, there were only enough beds for 1 percent of the city's Jewish residents.

---

40 Sroka, *Rada Miejska*, 290.

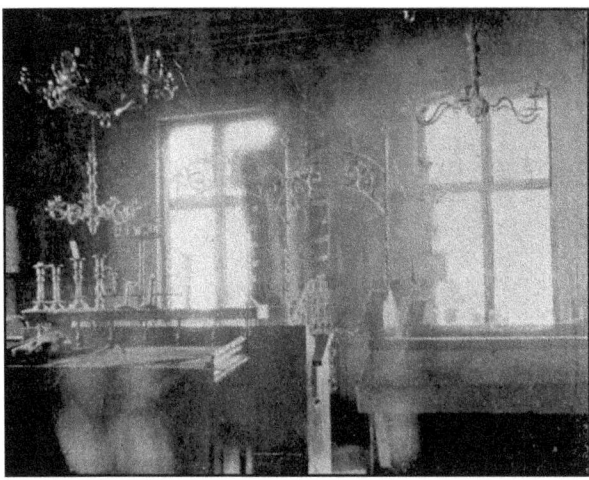

Figure 4.9. Hospital synagogue (before 1906). Mehrer, *Szpital lwowskiej gminy*, 49.

World War I

World War I affected the fate of the city, which had remained under Austro-Hungarian rule throughout the previous century. Lviv was occupied by Russian troops on the night of September 3–4, 1914. The city did not return to the Austro-Hungarian Empire until June 22, 1915, after the Battle of Gorlice and the Central Powers' counteroffensive.[41]

After the outbreak of the war, the Jewish Hospital faced new challenges. There was an influx of wounded and refugees to Lviv, and difficult living conditions contributed to the spread of diseases. It was necessary to provide medical care to all those in need, especially orphaned children. The Jewish Community began to organize an aid campaign through Jewish associations and organizations; the hospital was also involved. Increasingly stretched financially, the Jewish Community had less money with which to fund the hospital, and there were soon supplies shortages. The number of medical personnel also fluctuated, as doctors were called up for medical service in the Austrian army.[42] As a result, the hospital's activities were limited to the work of one department headed by Dr. Jan Landau.[43]

While most hospitals were used for military purposes, the Jewish Hospital escaped this fate, and during the Russian invasion part of it provided care for the mentally ill. Nevertheless, a number of hospital buildings were partially destroyed and there was a good deal of looting when the Russian troops left Lviv. For instance, they took bed linen with them.[44]

---

41 Józef Białynia-Chołodecki, *Lwów w czasie okupacji rosyjskiej (3 września 1914–22 czerwca 1915). Z własnych przeżyć i spostrzeżeń* (Lwów: nakł. Redakcji, 1930).
42 TsDIAL, fond 701, op. 3, spr. 686, f. 10.
43 TsDIAL, fond 701, op. 2, spr. 1779, f. 17–18, 22.
44 Feuerstein, *Trzydzieści lat*, 12.

Polish-Ukrainian war (1918–1919)

On November 1, 1918, with the fall of the Austro-Hungarian Empire, Ukrainian politicians proclaimed the establishment of the West Ukrainian People's Republic in Lviv and seized the city. The Polish population of Lviv, seeking to incorporate the city, as well as the entire territory of Eastern Galicia, into the Polish state reborn after partitions, opposed this with arms. This struggle between Lviv's Poles and Ukrainians developed into a full-blown Polish-Ukrainian war. After the Ukrainian army withdrew from Lviv, a pogrom against the Jewish population took place on November 22–23, 1918.[45]

The pogrom prompted the city's Jews to establish the Jewish Committee for Relief of Victims of Riots and Robberies in Lviv on November 29, 1918, also known as the Jewish Rescue Committee.[46] Chaired by Dr. Emil Parnas, Dr. Tobiasz Askenasy, and Dr. Rafał Buber, the committee had several dozen members recruited from among Lviv's Jewish intelligentsia. It offered emergency assistance to victims of the pogrom in the form of food, medical supplies, warm clothes, fuel, and nonrefundable loans. Uniting with other similar organizations, it eventually operated throughout Eastern Lesser Poland (Polish: Małopolska Wschodnia).

As early as December 2, 1918, the First Aid Section of the Jewish Rescue Committee was established, with the involvement of medical personnel from the Jewish Hospital. Members of the section—doctors and nurses, as well as medical students—provided medical aid to those wounded and sick and, if necessary, transported them to the hospital with the help of scouts. However, the hospital's activities were severely limited, as during the Polish-Ukrainian War both the hospital and adjacent buildings were further damaged (fig. 4.10). Equipment that had somehow survived World War I was also ruined.[47]

The early 1920s

World War I changed the course of Lviv's history. In November 1919, the Entente countries granted Poland a mandate over Eastern Galicia for a period of twenty-five years, which was converted a few years later into a permanent presence in the area. The Polish-Bolshevik War of 1919–1920 ended with the signing of a peace treaty in Riga on March 18, 1921. Under its terms, Lviv, along with all of Eastern Galicia, was to remain part of Poland.[48]

---

45 Grzegorz Gauden, *Lwów – kres iluzji: opowieść o pogromie listopadowym 1918* (Kraków: Towarzystwo Autorów i Wydawców Prac Naukowych Universitas, 2019); Wacław Wierzbieniec, "The Consequences of the Lviv Pogrom on November 22–23, 1918, in Light of the Findings and Actions of the Jewish Rescue Committee," *Scripta Judaica Cracoviensia* 18 (2020): 33–48.
46 Wierzbieniec, "The Consequences of the Lviv Pogrom."
47 Feuerstein, *Trzydzieści lat*, 12.
48 Lech Wyszczelski, *Wojna o Kresy Wschodnie 1918–1921* (Warsaw: Bellona, 2011).

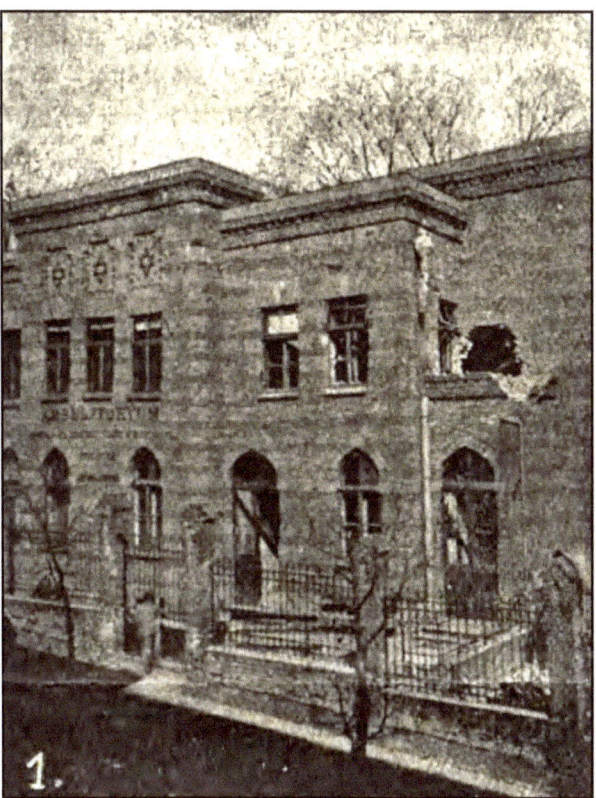

Figure 4.10. Damage to the facade of the hospital building (1919). *Nowości Ilustrowane*, no. 19 (1919): 5.

Lviv belonged to a group of large cities located on the territory of the Second Polish Republic and was the capital of the voivodship (in Polish: *województwo*). Despite its administrative role and position as an important cultural, scientific, and economic center, Lviv was not what it had been under the Austro-Hungarian Empire. Yet it remained the multiethnic and multidenominational city in which Jews had lived for centuries.

After the end of World War I, the health condition of Lviv residents was worse than poor. The highest mortality rates were in 1919, when 29.7 people per one thousand residents died.[49] Deteriorating housing and sanitary conditions were combined with a lack of adequate food and medical care. Epidemics of infectious diseases (especially typhoid) were also a serious problem. Epidemiological hospitals and bathhouses were developed in the city.[50] In November 1920, the Jewish Rescue Committee opened a bathing facility and a disinfection point at the Jewish Hospital. The latter could serve five hundred people a day and was the first facility of its kind in the city.[51] Measures to improve health and sanitary

---

49 Andrzej Bonusiak, *Lwów w latach 1918–1939. Ludność – Przestrzeń – Samorząd* (Rzeszów: Wydawnictwo Wyższej Szkoły Pedagogicznej, 2000), 252.
50 Ibid., 253.
51 TsDIAL, fond 505, op. 1, spr. 78, f. 16.

conditions in Lviv also included rebuilding and modernizing medical institutions, including the Jewish Hospital.

In 1919, the devastated hospital was placed under the leadership of Lviv-born Dr. Samuel Meisels, who set about repairing the infrastructure and replacing medical equipment. His task was made easier as he was also chair of the First Aid Section of the Jewish Rescue Committee.[52] The choice of Dr. Meisels as the hospital's director was no accident. He was a prominent pediatrician and social activist, committed to improving the lives of his fellow city residents.[53] He enjoyed widespread respect, and his position among Lviv physicians is evidenced by the fact that he remained in charge of the hospital throughout the interwar period. It is unknown what happened to him during World War II. His last publication, which appeared in 1939, was devoted to the importance of health services and hospitals during the war.[54]

The 1919 rebuilding of the hospital, and new laboratory and X-ray equipment, would not have been possible without the financial and in-kind support provided by the American Jewish Joint Distribution Committee (the JDC—also called Joint), an organization that was established in the United States in 1914 to aid Jews in Europe and Palestine.[55] The JDC dispersed medicines, clothing, food, hygiene supplies, and money for the repair and construction of hospitals, infirmaries, public baths and kitchens, orphanages, and health care infrastructure. It worked with schools to improve their sanitation and access to care and promoted hygiene and dental awareness. It also carried out campaigns against fascism.[56]

With the JDC's help, the Jewish Hospital was among the first three Lviv hospitals to resume operations; the others were the National General Hospital and the Hospital of the Sisters of Mercy. In addition, three Lviv sanatoriums run by doctors opened their doors again.[57]

Rebuilt and properly equipped, the Jewish Hospital gradually became an important major health care institution (fig. 4.11) once again. In the interwar period, it occupied six thousand square meters.[58] Gas lighting was replaced by electric lighting; water and sewage systems were expanded; and the number of toilets was increased and bathrooms with hot and cold water were installed in each ward. The hospital kitchen was rebuilt and expanded, and a new cold room was added. The hospital was one of the first medical centers in Lviv to have rubber and xylolite floors. It had equipment, including disinfecting apparatus,

---

52 Feuerstein, *Trzydzieści lat*, 13.
53 *Almanach żydowski*, 412.
54 Samuel Meisels, *Szpital a wojna nowoczesna* (Lwów: s.n.: 1939).
55 Feuerstein, *Trzydzieści lat*, 13.
56 See: Elissa Bemporad et al., *The JDC at 100: A Century of Humanitarianism* (Detroit: Wayne State University Press, 2019), ebook.
57 TsDIAL, fond 567, op. 1, spr. 44, f. 1.
58 "Szpital Izraelickiej Gminy Wyznaniowej Fundacji M. Lazarusa," in *Księga sanitarna m. Lwowa. Sprawozdanie z działalności Miejskiego Wydziału Zdrowia, instytucji i organizacji higieny publicznej za rok 1928 oraz rzut oka na rozwój stosunków sanitarnych w pierwszym dziesięcioleciu niepodległości państwa zebrał dr Eugeniusz Doliński, Naczelny Lekarz Miejski* (Lwów: nakładem Gminy Król. Stoł. Miasta Lwowa: 1929), 24.

some other Lviv institutions lacked.⁵⁹ Moreover, it had separate storage for linen, clothing, equipment, sanitary items, medicines, and food.⁶⁰

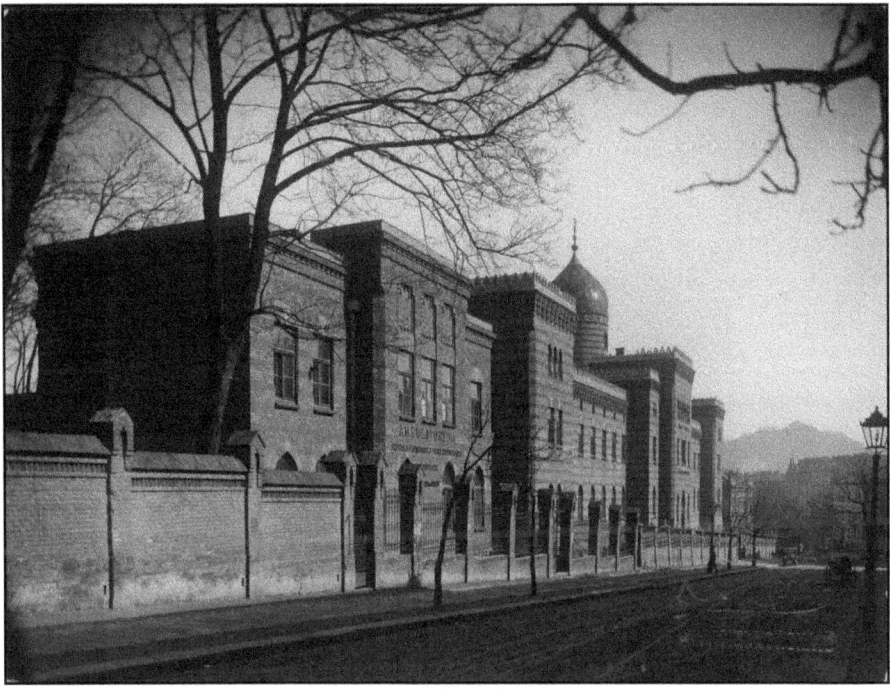

Figure 4.11. Jewish Hospital ca 1925. Photo: Marek Münz, BN, F.7819/II.

Improvements in the areas of disease treatment and prevention, mass vaccinations, diagnostics, and in the promotion of good nutrition and exercise soon saw results. Additionally, medical personal with better professional qualifications, physical education instructors, school- and summer-camp teachers, as well as the development of health education and prevention programs began to yield positive results, with great gains in the health of Lviv's population (219,388 people in 1921, including 76,854 Jews).⁶¹ In the following years, infectious diseases gave way to social diseases, such as tuberculosis, which in subsequent years were the cause of the largest number of deaths.⁶²

---

59 Feuerstein, *Trzydzieści lat*, 14.
60 TsDIAL, fond 701, op. 3, spr. 673, f. 14–16; fond 701, op. 3, spr. 861, f. 15–17; fond 701, op. 2, spr. 1779, f. 45–47.
61 Skorowidz miejscowości Rzeczypospolitej Polskiej: opracowany na podstawie wyników pierwszego powszechnego spisu ludności z dn. 30 września 1921 r. i innych źródeł urzędowych. T. 13, *Województwo lwowskie t. XII* (Warszawa: GUS, 1924), x.
62 Edyta Czop, "Stan zdrowotny ludności Lwowa w okresie międzywojennym (1918–1939)," in *L'viv: Misto – suspil'stwo – kul'tura, vol. 6, L'viv-Krakiv: dialoh mist v istorychnii retrospektyvi*, ed. Olena Arkusha and Marian Mudryi (L'viv: L'vivs'kyi Derzhavnyi Universytet imeni Ivana Franka, 2007), 511–522.

The rules guiding the Jewish Hospital in the interwar period

In addition to local and state government hospitals, in interwar period there were insurance-funded and private hospitals.[63] The rules of operation of public and private health care institutions—hospitals and outpatient clinics—were regulated by the March 22, 1928 Decree of the President of the Second Polish Republic on Medical Establishments.[64] The Jewish Hospital also operated under the rules established by the Jewish Community Council on January 5, 1927—the "Regulations for the Board of the Israelite Community Hospital in Lviv."[65]

While the hospital was the property of the Jewish Community Council, it served patients of all religions and offered care at least as good as that provided to the insured at public hospitals. It was unique in the way it fulfilled the religious needs of its Jewish patients. It functioned thanks to public subsidies, as well as funds from the Jewish community.[66] In the 1930s, the hospital was allowed to provide one-year internships for medical graduates.[67]

Hospital departments and outpatient clinics

The first departments to reopen after World War I were the surgical and internal medicine departments. Subsequently, other departments were created: pediatrics, pulmonology, neurology, urology, obstetrics, ophthalmology, otolaryngology, dermatology, and rheumatology.

In the interwar period, efforts were made to develop a multispecialty hospital which, as decreed by the Regulations for the Board of the Israelite Community Hospital in Lviv, included wards that provided around-the-clock care and outpatient clinics. The number of outpatient clinics varied, however. There were clinics for internal medicine, surgery, pediatrics, urology, dermatology, ENT, gynecology, ophthalmology, neurologhy, rheumatology, dentistry, cardiology, diabetes, and cancer testing and treatment (fig.4.12).[68]

In 1922, in the Old People's Home located next to the hospital, the Treatment Center for Children Sick with Favus (a chronic, inflammatory skin infection) was opened. The clinic had fifteen beds and was headed by Dr. Jakub Münzer.[69] In the same year, a department for children at risk of, or already suffering from, tuberculosis was opened. There was a terrace,

---

63 Eugeniusz Piestrzyński, *Dwadzieścia lat publicznej służby zdrowia w Polsce Odrodzonej: 1918–1938* (Warszawa: Ministerstwo Opieki Społecznej, 1939). Eugeniusz Sieńkowski, "Medycyna polska w okresie dwudziestolecia międzywojennego," *Nowiny Lekarskie*, no. 3 (1991): 60–66.
64 "Rozporządzenie Prezydenta Rzeczypospolitej z dnia 22 marca 1928 roku o zakładach leczniczych," in *Dziennik Ustaw RP* 1928, no 38, item 382.
65 TsDIAL, fond 701, op. 3, spr. 673, 1–24.
66 TsDIAL, fond 701, op. 4, spr. 313, f. 28; DALO, f. 1, op. 9, spr. 1523, f. 32.
67 TsDIAL, fond 701, op. 4, spr. 306, f. 60; fond 701, op. 3, spr. 1346, f. 2.
68 TsDIAL, fond 701, op. 3, spr. 1346, f. 2; Wiktor Chajes, *Sześć lat Żydowskiej Gminy Wyznaniowej* (Lwów: Wiktor Chajes, 1935), 24.
69 TsDIAL, fond 701, op. 2, spr. 1623, f. 33.

where children took therapeutic rests on sunny days.[70] The Jewish Hospital was the only place in Lviv that served children with tuberculosis, and in time it had most of the beds for tuberculosis patients in the city and the surrounding area.[71] In addition, the hospital had a pharmacy,[72] a light-therapy room, a chemical and bacteriological laboratory,[73] and an X-ray room.[74]

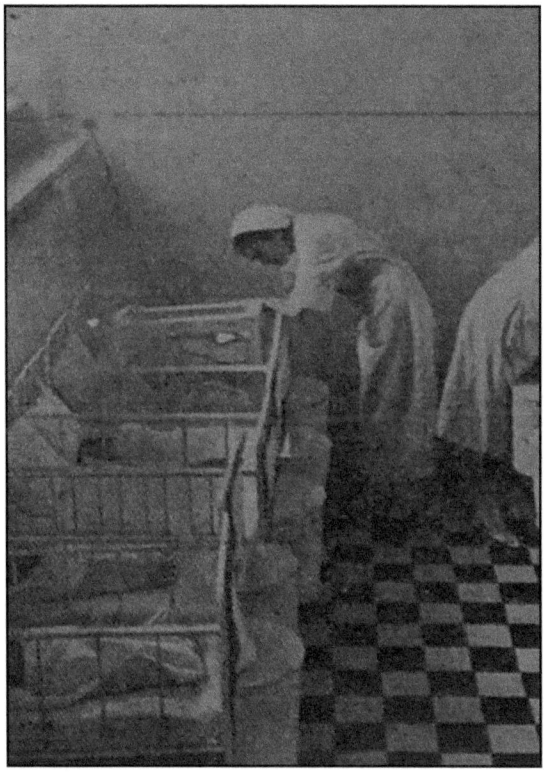

Figure 4.12. Room for newborns in the maternity department. *Almanach zdrowia TOZu i szpitala żydowskiego fundacji Maurycego Lazarusa* (Lwów: Wydawnictwo Kultura i Sztuka 1937), 13.

---

70 Ibid., f. 45, 59; TsDIAL, fond 701, op. 3, spr. 644, f. 18; "Otwarcie leżalni i oddziału światłoleczniczego," *Chwila* 1204 (1922): 6.

71 In 1937, the Internal Medicine Clinic of the Jan Kazimierz University had twenty-six beds for tuberculosis patients, the Social Security Hospital had forty-five, and the Laryngology Clinic, Internal Departments I and II, General Hospital had several beds. These beds were supplemented by forty beds at the Municipal Institution for Incurables on Janowska Street, seventy-five beds in post-sanatorium house, and 110 in the Holosko sanatorium; AAN, sygn. 2/15/0/-/1464, *Potrzeby w zakresie akcji przeciwgruźliczej na terenie m. Lwowa*, 1 X 1937 [w.f.].

72 DALO, fond 1, op. 9, spr. 523, f. 31.

73 TsDIAL, fond 503, op. 1, spr. 50, f. 88; fond 701, op. 3, spr. 673, f. 8; fond 701, op. 3, spr. 861, f. 9; fond 701, op. 2, spr. 1779, f. 39; "Rok pracy na niwie higieny. Z powodu rocznego zebrania Tow. szerz. higieny wśród Żydów," *Chwila* 2115 (1925): 6.

74 "Rok pracy na niwie higieny. Z powodu rocznego zebrania Tow. szerz. higieny wśród Żydów," *Chwila* 2115 (1925): 6.

Medical staff during the interwar period

In the interwar period, Lviv was one of the most important Jewish population centers in the Second Polish Republic. In 1921, 33 percent of Lviv's total population was of Jewish ancestry;[75] and between 1921 and 1931, the number of Lviv's Jews grew by 29.6 percent.[76] In the 1920s about eighty thousand Jews lived in the city. By 1931, Lviv was inhabited by 312,231 people, including 99,595 Jews,[77] accounting for 31.9 percent of the total population. This slight decrease in the city's percentage of Jews since 1921 was a result of the incorporation of suburban boroughs populated by non-Jews and creation of Greater Lviv.[78]

Lviv also saw a steady increase in the number of doctors. In 1922, 488 doctors were registered;[79] in 1930, there were 920 doctors working in the city; in 1931, there were 809;[80] and seven years later, there were 996.[81] Most of them were employed at the National General Hospital and the Jan Kazimierz University clinics (fig. 4.13).[82] In 1930, the latter boasted 153 doctors, 246 nurses, and 202 administrative and technical staff.[83]

The increase in the number of members of the Jewish community, and the resulting increased demand for health care, drove the Jewish Hospital's further growth. The hospital employed administrative staff, whose number remained constant throughout the interwar period and was limited to six people, in addition to technical staff, and medical staff.[84] The hospital ranked second in Lviv in medical personnel numbers. In 1931, there were seventeen doctors and thirty nurses; in 1937, there were twenty-nine doctors and forty-one nursing staff.[85]

The hospital employed Jews and non-Jews alike and the prewar department chairs—Dr. Pisek and Dr. Ruff—retained their positions. It employed doctors of both sexes, but men predominated. Lviv attracted women doctors because the city was more liberal than the countryside. While none of them became chief physician or department chair, they did head laboratories; for example, Dr. Ida Begleiter oversaw the chemical laboratory.[86]

---

75 *Skorowidz miejscowości*, x.
76 Piotr Trojański, "Liczba, rozmieszczenie oraz struktura wewnętrzna ludności wyznania mojżeszowego w województwie lwowskim w okresie międzywojnia," in Lwów. Miasto, społeczeństwo, kultura, t. II: *Studia z dziejów Lwowa*, ed. Henryk W. Żaliński and Kazimierz Karolczak (Kraków: Wydawnictwo Uniwersytetu Pedagogicznego: 1998), 249.
77 *Drugi powszechny spis ludności z dn. 9 XII 1931 r. Mieszkania i gospodarstwa domowe. Ludność. Stosunki zawodowe. Miasto Lwów* (Warszawa: GUS 1937), 11.
78 *Statystyka Polski*, series C, notebook 68 (Warszawa: GUS 1938), 36–40.
79 DALO, fond 1, op. 9, spr. 68, f. 41, 43; fond 1, op. 9, spr. 77, f. 45–72.
80 *Lwów w cyfrach: miesięcznik statystyczny/Léopol en chiffres: bulletin mensuel de statistique municipale* 1 (1931): 30.
81 Ibid.: 27–28.
82 Ibid.: 27.
83 Bonusiak, *Lwów w latach 1918–1939*, 256.
84 TsDIAL, fond 701, op. 3, spr. 1095, f. 12; fond 701, op. 4, spr. 304, f. 43–45, 46–50; fond 701, op. 4, spr. 306, f. 41–49; fond 701, op. 4, spr. 308, f. 35–42; fond 701 op. 4, spr. 314, f. 36–41, 44–46.
85 TsDIAL, fond 701, opis 4, spr. 304, f. 43–45, 46–50; fond 701, opis 4, spr. 314, f. 36–41, 44–46.
86 TsDIAL, fond 701, op. 3, spr. 1095, f. 12; fond 701, op. 4, spr. 304, f. 43–45, 46–50; fond 701, op. 4, spr. 306, f. 41–49; fond 701, op. 4, spr. 308, f. 35–42; fond 701, op. 4, spr. 314, f. 36–41, 44–46.

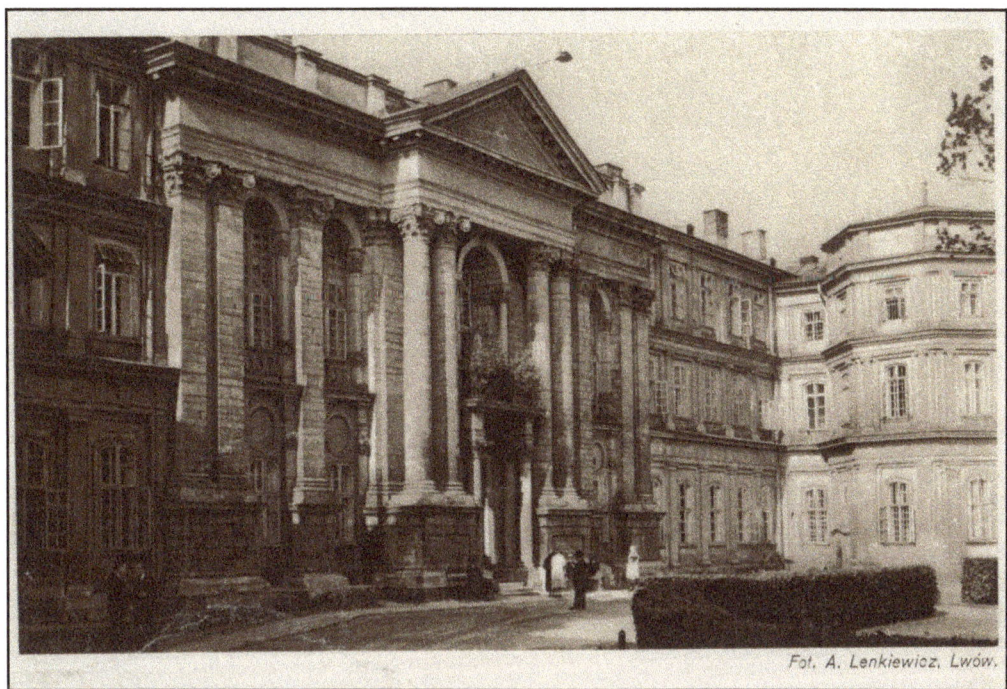

Figure 4.13. State General Hospital in Lviv (1937). "Lwów według zdjęć fotograficznych Adama Lenkiewicza" (Lwów: Nakład XV Zjazdu lekarzy i przyrodników polskich, 1937).

For the most part, the hospital's doctors came from assimilated homes, rather than from Orthodox backgrounds.[87] Interwar Lviv was one of only five cities in Poland where one could study medicine, which meant that many of the staff employed at the Jewish Hospital had trained in the city. Some, however, had studied abroad. As medical knowledge constantly developed, doctors at the hospital took internships or scholarships elsewhere in Poland or abroad. Some also practiced for many years in other cities. For example, Dr. Maria Oehlenberg (Öhlenberg), a specialist in internal and pediatric diseases, also practiced in Vienna.[88] Many also worked in spa towns during their vacations.

In Lviv, it was common for medical practitioners to occupy several positions. For instance, Dr. Samuel Lehm (1879–1954),[89] a laryngologist (fig. 4.14) and author of a number of articles on the subject, worked in the hospital's otolaryngology clinic, was a

---

87 One of the few representatives of the Orthodox Jewish community was Maximilian Ungar (b. 1903, Lviv), a graduate of the University of Prague, a specialist in heart and lung diseases, editor of the "Medical Calendar" and "Medicine and Health" sections of the Lviv-based *Chwila*, and a member of the TOZ; *Almanach żydowski*, 432–433.
88 TsDIAL, fond 503, op. 1, spr. 39, f. 79.
89 His son Stanisław Herman Lem (1921–2006) was a world-famous science fiction writer, the author of essays on various topics (including philosophy, futurology, and literary criticism), and a candidate for the Nobel Prize in Literature. He describes his childhood and school years spent in interwar Lviv in his autobiography *Wysoki Zamek* (High Castle).

doctor at the Social Insurance Institution in Lviv, and assisted Prof. Antoni Jurasz[90] in the Otolaryngology Polyclinic.[91] He ran his private practice as well. Other doctors at Jewish Hospital were also associated with the Faculty of Medicine at the Franciscan University of Lviv, renamed Jan Kazimierz University after the First World War.

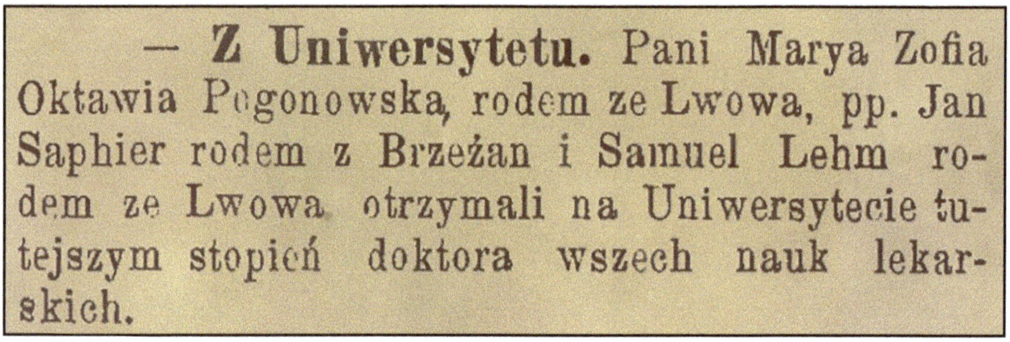

> — **Z Uniwersytetu.** Pani Marya Zofia Oktawia Pogonowska, rodem ze Lwowa, pp. Jan Saphier rodem z Brzeżan i Samuel Lehm rodem ze Lwowa otrzymali na Uniwersytecie tutejszym stopień doktora wszech nauk lekarskich.

Figure 4.14. Press release announcing that Samuel Lehm has graduated from the medical faculty at the Lviv University. *Gazeta Lwowska* 75 (1909): 3.

In the Second Polish Republic, physicians were organized into three types of associations: general and specialized scientific societies (national and regional, single- or multifaith), the self-governing Lviv Association of Physicians, and professional associations. In Lviv there were, among others, the Society of Polish Physicians, the Lviv Medical Society, the Lviv Regional Association of Physicians of the Polish State, the Association of Physicians of the Republic of Poland, and the Association of Physicians of the National Health Fund in Lviv. Bringing together doctors of different faiths, these organizations advanced and promoted medical science by organizing lectures and running libraries. There were also societies for different minorities—for example, the Ukrainian Medical Society and the (Jewish) Circle of TOZ Doctors.[92] Among the leading members of these societies were doctors who worked at the Jewish Hospital: Dr. Arnold Schwarz (dermatology), for instance, was vice-president of the Circle of TOZ Doctors and was a doctor at the Lviv Health Care Society for many years.

During the interwar period, the Circle of TOZ Doctors was active at the Jewish Hospital, where they increased their knowledge through regular lectures.[93] Since tuberculosis was the biggest social health problem, Jewish doctors became involved in the societies dedicated

---

90 Antoni Jurasz (1847–1923), a Polish otolaryngologist associated with the Universities of Heidelberg, Lviv, and Poznan, pioneered work in the field of rhinoscopy. He is credited with the invention of many medical instruments used in the field of rhinolaryngology, including a specialized tool called d nasopharyngeal forceps.
91 Gajewska Agnieszka, *Wypędzony z Wysokiego Zamku. Biografia* (Warsaw: Wydawnictwo Literackie, 2021).
92 It was established in March 1936 on the initiative of Dr. Natan Aron Schneider, mentioned in the first chapter of this book. Its main goal was to engage physicians in the scientific and social fields. For this reason, lectures, readings, and speeches, as well as discussions on practical and theoretical medicine were arranged for colleagues living in Lviv and its surrounds.
93 Jakimyszyn-Gadocha, *W trosce o zdrowie*, 216.

to fighting it. The most active member of this group was Dr. Marcin Selzer, head of the tuberculosis sanatorium in Holosko and the founder and head of the TOZ anti-tuberculosis clinic.[94] Doctors were also involved in Jewish and non-Jewish philanthropic and cultural organizations.

Several doctors employed at the Jewish Hospital took part in the First World War. In the Austro-Hungarian Empire, Universal mobilization began on July 30, 1914. Doctors were given officer ranks. The head of the women's surgical department, Dr. Aron Wolf (b. 1876), and the head of the pediatric surgery department, Dr. Jakub Münzer (b. 1872), were awarded the Signum Laudis, a medal given to officers for outstanding military service to the Austro-Hungarian Empire in both peace and war.[95] The long-time head of the men's surgical department, Dr. Samuel Oberländer (b. 1880), was chief physician at the Citadel (a complex of fortifications built in the mid-nineteenth century) in Lviv, commandant of the hospital in Radymno, and head of the garrison surgical hospital department in Lviv;[96] and Dr. Alexander Rosenberg (b. 1886), who worked in the Gynecological Clinic, was commandant of Field Military Hospital no. 305.[97] Some doctors also participated in the Polish-Bolshevik War. One of them was Otto Finsterbusch (b. 1898), a gynecologist (surgeon) at the National General Hospital and the Jewish Hospital, and member of the Gynecological Society in Lviv.[98]

Jewish Hospital doctors were also represented in the Sejm of the Second Polish Republic. Dr. Aron Wolf, for instance, a Zionist since his early youth, was a member of Sejm in 1929–1930.

Nurses—that is, members of the lower-level medical staff—were almost always women.[99] Their tasks included administering medicines and meals, changing linen, following doctors' orders, preparing patients for appointments and procedures, and maintaining order in operating rooms and patients' rooms. Nurses were assisted by girls training for the profession.[100]

---

94 *Almanach żydowski*, 427–428.
95 Ibid., 439–440, 518–519.
96 Ibid., 414–415.
97 Ibid., 254–255.
98 Ibid., 384–385.
99 TsDIAL, fond 701, op. 3, spr. 1095, f. 12; fond 701, op. 4, spr. 304, f. 43–45, 46–50; fond 701, op. 4, spr. 306, f. 41–49; fond 701, op. 4, spr. 308, f. 35–42; fond 701, op. 4, spr. 314, f. 36–41, 44–46.
100 TsDIAL, fond 701, op. 3, spr. 673, f. 8; fond 701, op. 3, spr. 861, f. 9; fond 701, op. 2, spr. 1779, f. 39.

Statistics

In 1919, the hospital had one hundred beds. As the years passed, the number increased: 115 in 1922;[101] 131 in 1924;[102] and 140 in 1927–1928.[103] In the 1930s, the number of beds ranged from 130 to 188,[104] and the Jewish Hospital ranked second among Lviv institutions (the National General Hospital with clinics of Jan Kazimierz University had 1,511 beds between them).[105] The number of beds in the Jewish Hospital, however, did not correspond to the actual needs of the Jewish population of the city. Indeed, there was one hospital bed per thousand Jews living in Lviv in 1931, while in the entire city, with a total of 3,506 beds, there were six beds per thousand residents.[106] This state of affairs—despite the relatively large number of Lviv hospitals—did not deviate from the standards of the time. Depending on the region, there was anything between a handful and several dozen beds per ten thousand residents in the Second Polish Republic.[107] Complete data on the number of patients at the Jewish Hospital during the interwar period has not survived. However, between 1929 and 1933, there was an increase from 1,400 to more than 2,400 per year.[108]

Before the outbreak of World War I, up to twenty thousand people a year were admitted to hospital outpatient clinics.[109] Between the wars, the number of outpatient consultations increased from more than 37,000 (1929) to more than 45,000 (1933). In subsequent years, the number reached fifty thousand,[110] the two oldest outpatient clinics—internal medicine and surgery—being the most popular.

The hospital is still active today, 120 years after its inauguration, presently as a municipal maternity hospital (fig. 4.15).

---

101 DALO, fond 1, op. 9, spr. 81, f. 67.
102 DALO, fond 1, op. 9, spr. 457, f. 15, 123; fond 1, op. 9, spr. 1523, f. 78.
103 *Lwów w cyfrach: miesięcznik statystyczny/Léopol en chiffres: bulletin mensuel de statistique municipale*, 4 (1932), 28.
104 AAN, sign. 2/15/0/-/806, f. 40.
105 *Lwów w cyfrach* 4 (1932): 28.
106 Ibid.
107 Piotr Grata, *Polityka społeczna Drugiej Rzeczypospolitej: uwarunkowania, instytucje, działania* (Rzeszów: Wydawnictwo Uniwersytetu Rzeszowskiego, 2013), 278.
108 TsDIAL, fond 701, op. 3, spr. 1346, f. 2.
109 DALO, fond 2, op. 1, spr. 3062, f. 50.
110 Chajes, *Sześć lat*, 24; Feuerstein, *Trzydzieści lat szpitala* 14.

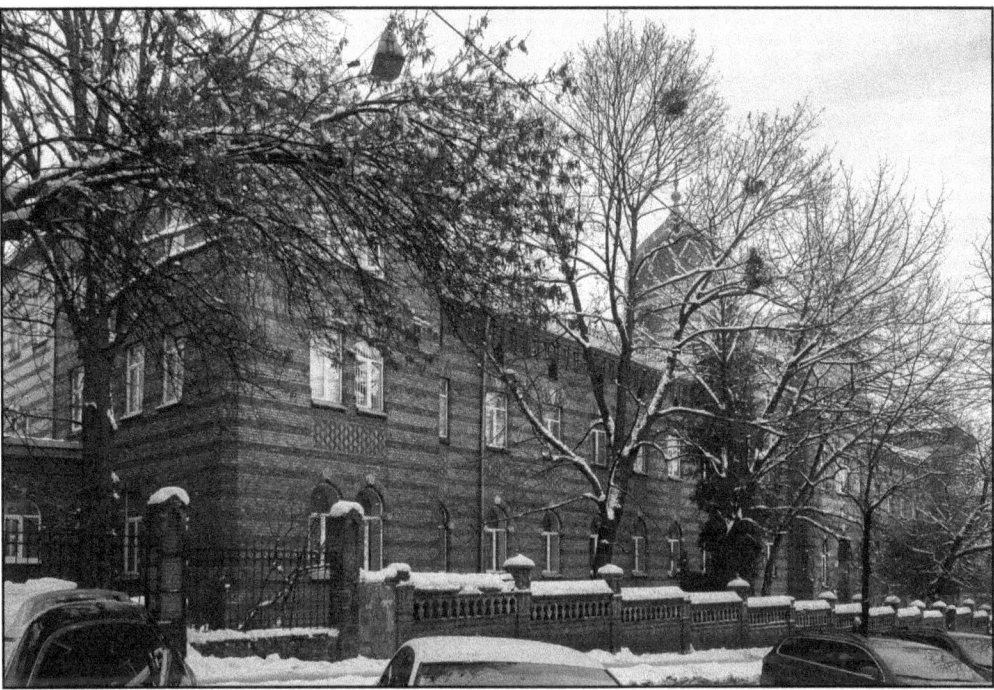

Figure 4.15. View of the former Jewish Hospital from the southwest, Photo: Olha Zarechnyuk, December 2023.

***

As already mentioned, the Jewish Hospital was established to help all the sick, regardless of religion or background. As the hospital was a religious institution, it was dominated by Jewish patients. However, the comprehensive care available, modern equipment, and the possibility of obtaining free or partially paid assistance attracted patients from other religions and of various nationalities. Equally important were the qualifications and experience of the doctors working there. These physicians had studied at the best universities (primarily in Vienna, Kraków, and Lviv), taken the most prestigious foreign internships, and were familiar with the latest scientific discoveries and treatment methods. Due to the fact that its physicians were members of both Polish and foreign medical associations, published research in professional journals, advanced science, and were involved in educating the population of Lviv about medicine and hygiene,[111] it is no surprise that the Jewish Hospital was held in such high esteem.

---

111 My work on the biographies of doctors working at the hospital is in preparation.

Archival Sources

ANK
Sign. ABM 42, district VIII, 1, f. 37.

AAN
Sign. 2/15/0/-/806, f. 40; 2/15/0/-/1464 [w.f.].

DALO
Fond 1, op. 9, spr. 68, f. 41, 43; fond 1, op. 9, spr. 77, f. 45–72; fond 1, op. 9, spr. 81, f. 67; fond 1, op. 9, spr. 457, f. 15, 123; fond 1, op. 9, spr. 523, f. 31; fond 1, op. 9, spr. 1523, f. 23, 78.
Fond 2, op. 1, spr. 3062, f. 50.

TsDIAL
Fond 503, op. 1, spr. 39, f. 79; fond 503, op. 1, spr. 50, f. 88; fond 505, op. 1, spr. 78, f. 16; fond 567, op. 1, spr. 44, f. 1.
Fond 701, op. 2, spr. 1559, f. 50–59; fond 701, op. 2., spr. 1623, f. 33; fond 701, op. 2, spr. 1779, f. 17–18, 22, 39, 45–47.
Fond 701, op. 3, spr. 644, f. 18; fond 701, op. 3, spr. 673, f. f. 1–24; fond 701, op. 3, spr. 686, f. 10; fond 701, op. 3, spr. 861, f. 9, 15–17; fond 701, op. 3, spr. 873, f. 28; fond 701, op. 3, spr. 1095, f. 12; fond 701, op. 3, spr. 1346, f. 2.
Fond 701, op. 4, spr. 304, f. 43–45, 46–50; fond 701, op. 4, spr. 306, f. 41–49, 60; fond 701, op. 4, spr. 308, f. 35–42; fond 701, op. 4, spr. 313, f. 28; fond 701, op. 4, spr. 314, f. f. 36–41, 44–46.

Bibliography

Almanach żydowski wydany przez Hermana Stachla zawierający szereg artykułów wybitnych literatów, polityków i publicystów oraz życiorysy czołowych postaci Małopolski Wschodniej. Lwów: Wydawnictwo Kultura i Sztuka, 1937.
Bemporad, Elissa, Jaclyn Granick, Suzanne D. Rutland, Veerle Vanden Daelen, Avinoam J. Patt, Atina Grossmann, Linda G. Levi, and Maud Mandel. *The JDC at 100: A Century of Humanitarianism*. Detroit: Wayne State University Press, 2019. Ebook.
Białynia-Chołodecki, Józef. *Lwów w czasie okupacji rosyjskiej (3 września 1914–22 czerwca 1915). Z własnych przeżyć i spostrzeżeń.* Lwów: nakł. Redakcji, 1930.
Bridgman, Robert Frédéric. *L'hôpital et la Cité.* Paris: Editions du Cosmos, 1963.
Bonusiak, Andrzej. *Lwów w latach 1918–1939. Ludność – Przestrzeń – Samorząd.* Rzeszów: Wydawnictwo Wyższej Szkoły Pedagogicznej, 2000.
Broński, Krzysztof. "Galicja w dobie autonomii wobec wyzwań nowoczesności." In *Między zacofaniem a modernizacją. Społeczno-gospodarcze problemy ziem polskich*

na przestrzeni wieków, edited by Elżbieta Kościk and Tomasz Głowiński, 395–412. Wrocław: Gajt Wydawnictwo, 2009.

Chajes, Wiktor. *Sześć lat Żydowskiej Gminy Wyznaniowej*. Lwów: Wiktor Chajes, 1935.

Czop, Edyta. "Stan zdrowotny ludności Lwowa w okresie międzywojennym (1918–1939)." In *Lwiw: misto – suspilstwo – kultura*. Vol. 6, Lwiw-Krakiw: dialog mist w istoričnìej retrospektiwi, edited by Olena Arkusza and Marian Mudrowo, 511–522. Lwiw: Lvìvskij Deržavnij Unìversitet ìmeni Ìvana Franka, 2007.

Drugi powszechny spis ludności z dn. 9 XII 1931 r. Mieszkania i gospodarstwa domowe. Ludność. Stosunki zawodowe. Miasto Lwów. Warszawa: GUS, 1937.

Dybiec, Julian. "Galicja na drodze do wielkiej przemiany." In *Kraków i Galicja wobec przemian cywilizacyjnych (1866–1914). Studia i szkice*, edited by Krzysztof Fiołek and Marian Stala, 31–42. Kraków: Towarzystwo Autorów i Wydawców Prac Naukowych Universitas, 2011.

———. "Nauka a modernizacja społeczna w Galicji w epoce autonomii." In *Galicja i jej dziedzictwo, t. 20: Historia wychowania, misja i edukacja*, edited by Kazimierz Szmyd and Julian Dybiec, 58–65. Rzeszów: Wydawnictwo Uniwersytetu Rzeszowskiego, 2008.

Feuerstein, Henryk. "Trzydzieści lat szpitala fundacji błp. Maurycego Lazarusa (Reportaż ze wspomnień, cyfr i faktów)." In *Almanach zdrowia TOZ-u i Szpitala Żydowskiego fundacji Maurycego Lazarusa*, 10–15. Lwów: TOZ, 1937.

Franaszek, Piotr. "Krajowy szpital powszechny we Lwowie na przełomie XIX i XX wieku." *Zeszyty naukowe Uniwersytetu Jagiellońskiego: Prace historyczne* 127 (2000): 121–135.

———. *Zdrowie publiczne w Galicji w dobie autonomii (Wybrane problemy)*. Kraków: Wydawnictwo Uniwersytetu Jagiellońskiego, 2002.

Gajewska, Agnieszka. *Wypędzony z Wysokiego Zamku. Biografia*. Warsaw: Wydawnictwo Literackie, 2021.

Gauden, Grzegorz. *Lwów – kres iluzji: opowieść o pogromie listopadowym 1918*. Kraków: Towarzystwo Autorów i Wydawców Prac Naukowych Universitas, 2019.

Grata, Piotr. *Polityka społeczna Drugiej Rzeczypospolitej: uwarunkowania, instytucje, działania*. Rzeszów: Wydawnictwo Uniwersytetu Rzeszowskiego, 2013.

Meisels, Samuel. *Szpital a wojna nowoczesna*. Lwów: n.p., 1939.

Heindl, Michael, and Ruth Koblizek. *125 Jahre Rothschild-Spital*. Wien: Dagobert Wien, 1998.

Jakimyszyn, Anna. *Żydzi krakowscy w dobie Rzeczypospolitej Krakowskiej: status prawny, przeobrażenia gminy, system edukacyjny*. Kraków: Wydawnictwo Austeria, 2008.

Jakimyszyn-Gadocha, Anna. *W trosce o zdrowie żydowskiej społeczności Lwowa (1918–1939)*. Kraków: Wydawnictwo Austeria, 2021.

Kitsera, Oleksandr. "Mytropolyt Andrey Sheptyts'kyy i 'Narodna lichnytsya.'" *Likars'kyy zbirnyk. Nova seriya* 13 (2004): 66–74.

Krętowski, Józef. *Ich pamięci... Straty osobowe lekarzy na Kresach Rzeczypospolitej w latach drugiej wojny światowej*. Białystok: Skryba, 2018.

Lwów w cyfrach: miesięcznik statystyczny/Léopol en chiffres: bulletin mensuel de statistique municipale 1 (1931); 4 (1932).

Nataliya Matlashenko. "Narodna lichnytsya – persha ukrayinska likarnya v Halychyni." *Farmatsevt praktyk* (2015). http://fp.com.ua/articles/ narodna-lichnitsya-persha-ukrayinska-likarnya-v-galichini.

Mehrer, Henryk. *Szpital lwowskiej gminy wyznaniowej izraelickiej fundacyi Maurycego Lazarusa*. Lwów: Szpital Lwowskiej Gminy Wyzn. Izraelickiej, 1906.

Organisations-Statut fuer das Spital der Israelitischen Kultusgemeinde in Wien. Wien: Selbstverlage der Direction, 1871.

Ostrowska, Teresa. "Stanisław Ruff." In *Polski Słownik Biograficzny* (Wrocław: Zakład Narodowy im. Ossolińskich – Wydawnictwo Polskiej Akademii Nauk, 1991).

"Otwarcie leżalni i oddziału światło leczniczego." *Chwila* 1204 (1922): 6.

Pawlikowski, Antoni. "Stosunki zdrowotne." In *Miasto Lwów w okresie samorządu 1870–1895*, edited by Edmund Mochnacki, 269–271. Lwów: Z drukarni W. A. Szyjkowskiego nakł. Gminy Król. Stoł. Miasta Lwowa, 1896.

Piestrzyński, Eugeniusz. *Dwadzieścia lat publicznej służby zdrowia w Polsce Odrodzonej: 1918–1938*. Warszawa: Ministerstwo Opieki Społecznej, 1939.

Purchla, Jacek. "Kraków i Lwów: zmienność relacji w XIX i XX wieku." In *Kraków i Lwów w cywilizacji europejskiej: materiały międzynarodowej konferencji zorganizowanej w dniach 15–16 listopada 2002*, edited by Jacek Purchla and Marta Dyhas, 81–90. Kraków: Międzynarodowe Centrum Kultury, 2003.

"Rok pracy na niwie higieny. Z powodu rocznego zebrania Tow. szerz. higieny wśród Żydów." *Chwila* 2115 (1925): 6.

"Rozporządzenie Prezydenta Rzeczypospolitej z dnia 22 marca 1928 roku o zakładach leczniczych." In *Dziennik Ustaw RP* 1928, no 38, item 382.

Sieńkowski, Eugeniusz. "Medycyna polska w okresie dwudziestolecia międzywojennego," *Nowiny Lekarskie* no. 3 (1991), 60–66.

Skorowidz miejscowości Rzeczypospolitej Polskiej: opracowany na podstawie wyników pierwszego powszechnego spisu ludności z dn. 30 września 1921 r. i innych źródeł urzędowych. T. 13, Województwo lwowskie t. XII. Warszawa: GUS, 1924.

Skotnicki, Aleksander B. *Szpital Gminy Wyznaniowej Żydowskiej w Krakowie 1866–1941*. Kraków: Stradomskie Centrum Dialogu, 2013.

Sroka, Łukasz T. *In the Light of Vienna: Jews in Lviv—between Tradition and Modernisation (1867–1914)*. Berlin: Peter Lang, 2018.

———. *Rada Miejska we Lwowie w okresie autonomii galicyjskiej 1870–1914. Studium o elicie władzy*. Kraków: Wydawnictwo Naukowe Uniwersytetu Pedagogicznego, 2012.

———. "Zaangażowanie społeczne elit żydowskich we Lwowie w okresie autonomii galicyjskiej." In *L'viv: Misto – suspil'stvo – kul'tura. Vol. 8, Chastyna 1: Vlada i suspil'stvo*, edited by Olena Arkusha and Marian Mudryi, 351–364. L'viv: L'vivs'kyi Derzhavnyi Universytet imeni Ivana Franka, 2012.

Statystyka Polski. Series C, notebook 68. Warszawa: GUS, 1938.

Strojnowski, Jerzy. "Józef Oettinger, pierwszy habilitowany docent i profesor historii medycyny na polskim uniwersytecie." *Kwartalnik Historii Nauki i Techniki* 15 (1970): 57–69.

"Szpital Izraelickiej Gminy Wyznaniowej Fundacji M. Lazarusa." In *Księga sanitarna m. Lwowa. Sprawozdanie z działalności Miejskiego Wydziału Zdrowia, instytucji i organizacji higieny publicznej za rok 1928 oraz rzut oka na rozwój stosunków sanitarnych w pierwszym dziesięcioleciu niepodległości państwa zebrał dr Eugeniusz Doliński, Naczelny Lekarz Miejski.* Lwów: nakładem Gminy Król. Stoł. Miasta Lwowa: 1929.

Trojański, Piotr. "Liczba, rozmieszczenie oraz struktura wewnętrzna ludności wyznania mojżeszowego w województwie lwowskim w okresie międzywojnia." In Lwów. Miasto, społeczeństwo, kultura. Vol. 2, *Studia z dziejów Lwowa*, edited by Henryk W. Żaliński and Kazimierz Karolczak, 243–260. Kraków: Wydawnictwo Uniwersytetu Pedagogicznego, 1998.

Waszczyszyn, Elżbieta. "The Changes in 19th Century European Hospital Architecture. Selected Examples." *Technical Transactions Architecture* 3-A (2015): 179–203.

Wierzbieniec, Wacław. "The Consequences of the Lviv Pogrom on November 22–23, 1918, in Light of the Findings and Actions of the Jewish Rescue Committee." *Scripta Judaica Cracoviensia* 18 (2020): 33–48.

Wnęk, Konrad. "Przemiany demograficzne we Lwowie w latach 1829–1938." *Zeszyty Naukowe Uniwersytetu Jagiellońskiego. Prace Historyczne* 135 (2008): 113–127.

Wnęk, Konrad, Lidia A. Zyblikiewicz, and Ewa Callahan. *Ludność nowoczesnego Lwowa w latach 1857–1938.* Kraków: Tow. Nauk. Societas Vistulana, 2006.

Wölfler, Bernhard. *Das alte und neue Wiener Israeliten-Spital nach authentischen Quellen dargestellt.* Wien: Gerold, 1873.

Wyszczelski, Lech. *Wojna o Kresy Wschodnie 1918–1921.* Warsaw: Bellona, 2011.

Zbroja, Barbara. *Miasto umarłych: architektura publiczna Żydowskiej Gminy Wyznaniowej w Krakowie w latach 1868–1939.* Kraków: Wydawnictwo WAM, 2005.

Postscript

The former Jewish Hospital has been in use by the inhabitants of Lviv for 120 years. While the borders have changed several times, as well as the language spoken in the city, its mission to serve people of this city has stayed the same. It is the legacy of Maurycy Lazarus, the great philanthropist of Lviv.

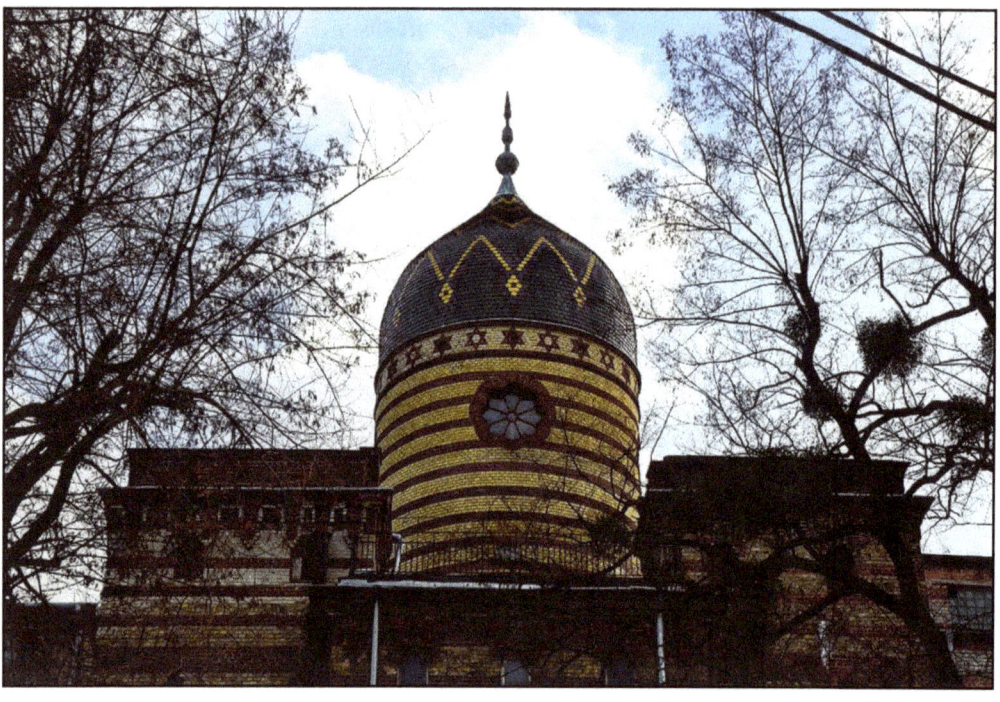

Figure 5.1. Jewish Hospital in Lviv. Wikimedia.[1] Photo: E. Lviv, November 2022.

---

1 Under Creative Commons license: https://creativecommons.org/licenses/by-sa/4.0/.

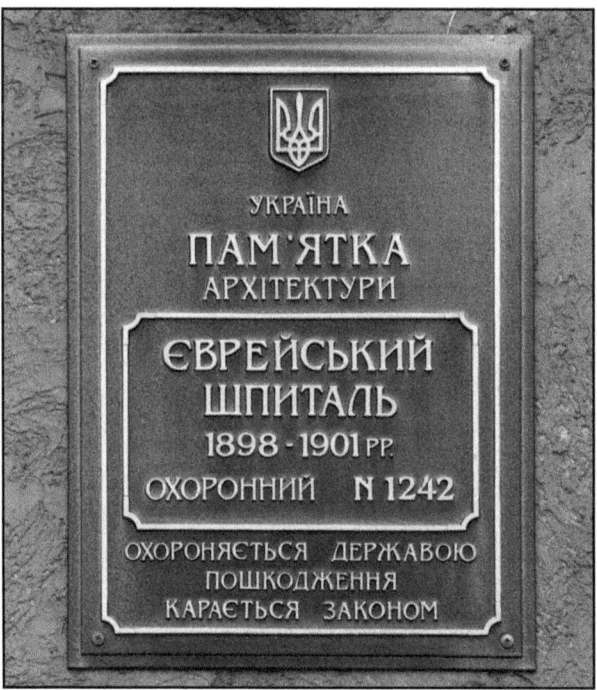

Figure 5.2. Commemorative plaque on the hospital wall. Photo: Olha Zarechnyuk, December 2023. (Translation from Ukrainian: Ukraine. Architectural landmark number 1242. The Jewish Hospital, 1898–1901. Under state preservation, damage is punishable by law.)

Contributors

Ewa Herbst, PhD is a great-granddaughter of Maurycy Lazarus, the founder of the Jewish Hospital in Lviv. She is an electrical and biomedical engineer, a former visiting professor at the University of Kentucky in Lexington and at Tulane University in New Orleans, principal research engineer at a biomedical instrument company, as well as CEO of her own research and development firm. In addition to publications in her area of research and several patents, she is the author of the book *Dokument podróży* (Travel Document), a story in poems and prose of her emotional turmoil after being forced out of Poland as a result of the wave of antisemitism that swept the country in 1967–69. She is also the author of "Herman Diamand—on the 90th Anniversary of His Death" (*Kwartalnik Historii Żydów/Jewish History Quarterly*, 287, no. 3 [2023]), an article about her great-uncle, one of the leading Galician and Polish politicians.

Anna Jakimyszyn-Gadocha, Dr. habil. (Institute of Jewish Studies, Jagiellonian University, Kraków) is a historian and a specialist in Judaic studies, and author of the following books: *Żydzi krakowscy w dobie Rzeczypospolitej Krakowskiej. Status prawny. Przeobrażenia gminy. System edukacyjny* (2008), *Mykwa. Dzieje żydowskiej łaźni rytualnej przy ul. Szerokiej w Krakowie* (2012), *Yiddish-English-Polish Dictionary* (2016), *W trosce o zdrowie żydowskiej społeczności Lwowa (1918–1939)* (2021), and numerous articles. She is also the translator of *Statut krakowskiej gminy żydowskiej z 1595 roku i jego uzupełnienia* (2005). She is the co-editor of ממרא דפולין *Mamre de-Polin. Księga jubileuszowa dedykowana Profesorowi Edwardowi Dąbrowie* (2021) and of Anna Rutkowski's Polish translation of *Memoirs of Glickl of Hammeln* (*Glikl. Siedem ksiąg. Pamiętniki z lat 1691–1719* (2021).

Sergey R. Kravtsov, PhD is a research fellow at the Center for Jewish Art, Hebrew University of Jerusalem. Born in Lviv, Ukraine, he was trained as an architect in his native city. In 1993, he received his doctoral degree from the Institute for the Theory and History of Architecture in Moscow, and moved to Israel in 1994. His research areas are the history of town planning, architectural theory, and the history of synagogue architecture. He is the author of *Di Gildene Royze: The Turei Zahav Synagogue in L'viv* (2011) and *In the Shadow of Empires: Synagogue Architecture in East-Central Europe* (2018), and a co-author of *Synagogues in Lithuania: A Catalogue* (2010–2012) and *Synagogues in Ukraine: Volhynia* (2017). He has also published about ninety essays in his research areas and edited and co-edited three books.

Andrew Zalewski, MD is a physician and former professor of medicine at Thomas Jefferson University in Philadelphia. He has authored two books on Austrian Galicia: *Galician Trails: The Forgotten Story of One Family* (2012) and *Galician Portraits: In Search of Jewish Roots* (2014), both of which reconstruct the story of his ancestors in a broader historical context. As the vice president of Gesher Galicia, he led archival research on Jewish educational access, in part supported by a grant from the Republic of Austria. His writings focus on Jewish cultural transformation, the impact of Jewish physicians, and Jewish legal rights in Galicia.

Dr. Zalewski is a frequent speaker at cultural and academic institutions in the US and abroad. His Gratz College course on the Jews of Galicia examines the internal and external forces behind the Jewish path to modernity. Unique archival records provide the background for his in-depth description of multiethnic Galicia.

Index

Page numbers in italics refer to figures and table.

A
Abigdor, Abraham, 5n11
Ackord, Abraham Samuel, 13n29
Arzt, Moses, 16n34
Ashkenazi, Solomon, 4
Askenasy, Tobiasz, 138

B
Ba'al Shem, Hillel, 9n18
Badenis, counts, 55
Barach, Adam (Ascher), 17, 23, 25–27, 34
Barach-Rappaport, Adam. *See* Barach, Adam
Barth, Wolf, 16n34
Bebel, August, 73
Begleiter, Ida, 144
Berger, Salomon Ber, 96
Bersohn, Matthias, 117
Bona Sforza, queen, 4
Borkowski, Mieczysław, count, 55
Borrel, Amédée, 75
Braun, Cecilia, 31
Buber, Rafał, 138
Buber, Szaja Abraham, 96
Byk, Emil, 60, 97

C
Calahora, Aron, 3
Calahora (Kalahora), Salomon, *3*, 4
Caro, Jecheskiel, 118
Caro, Joseph, 118
Cases, Joseph, 8n16
Casimir III the Great, king, 91–92

Chipiez, Charles, 113
Chmielowski, Albert, 110n41
Conegliano, Solomon, 8n16
Curie, Marie (*née* Skłodowska), 75

D
Daniel, king, 90
DeJona, Emanuel (Simcha Menachem), 4–5
Delmedigo, Joseph, 2n2
Diamand, Aleksander, 78–80
Diamand, Betti, 78
Diamand, Eleonora (*née* Lazarus, wife of Aleksander Diamand), 73, 75, 76–77, 78–80, 81
Diamand, Herman, 71, 74–75, 78, 79, 82n122
Diamand Hermina (*née* Lazarus, wife of Herman Diamand), 73-75
Diamand, Maurycy (father of Aleksander and Herman), 71, 78
Donhajser-Sikorska, Helena, 33n69
Dubs, Lazar, 25n53
Dzięcioł, Józefa, *82*
Dzieduszycki, Włodzimierz, 54

E
Eder, Józef, *54, 70*
Ehrlich, Dawid, 133–35
Ekielski, Władysław, 113
Epstein, Dina (*née* Waringer), 25
Epstein, Isaac, 17, 23–25, 27, 34
Epstein, Lea. *See* Mahl, Lea
Epstein, Mayer, 23
Ergas, Sofie. *See* Lazarus, Sofie

Erter, Isaac, 17n37

F
Falska, Maryna, 81
Felińska, Aniela (*née* Baurowicz), 119
Feliński, Feliks, 119
Feliński, Roman, *119–21*
Felix, Gabriel, 5, 8n12
Ferdinand, emperor, 50
Finsterbusch, Otto, 147
Fleck, Isidor (Eisig), 103
Fleck, Ludwik, 103n20
Fleck, Maurycy (Yitzhak Moshe), 103
Fleischer, Max, 113
Fleischl, Antoni Rudolf, 96
Förster, Ludwig, 107–9
Fortis, Abraham Isaac, 4
Fortis, Moses, 5n8
Franz Joseph I, emperor, 22, 30, 42, 53, 58, 61, 94, 108, 113, 130
Fröschel, Salomon Benjamin, 14, *15*
Fuchs, Franciszka. *See* Reich, Franciszka

G
Gartner, Jacob, 113
Geiger, Abraham, 104
Godowski, Władysław, 100
Goldszmit, Henryk. *See* Korczak, Janusz
Gołuchowski, Stanisław, 54
Gordons, medical family, 5
Graetz, Heinrich, 104
Gysis, Nikolaus, 103n21

H
Hansen, Theophilus, 107–9, 112
Hawryszkiewicz, Sylwester, 108n31
Henner, J. (Jakub), *70*
Herzl, Theodor, 71
Hirsch, Maurice (Maurycy) de, baron, 60–61
Hispanus, Isaac, 2
Hlávka, Josef, 112
Hochberger, Juliusz, 109–11, *113*, 120
Holzer, Wilhelm, 65
Homberg, Herz, 47, 49–50
Honigsmann, Oswald, 60
Horowitz, Maria, 33n69
Horowitz, Samuel, 56, 61, 66

J
Jeiteles, Jonas, 13
John Paul II, pope, 110n41
Jolles, Caroline (mother of Róża Maria), 52
Jolles, Róża Maria (Rosa Marie). *See* Lazarus, Róża Maria
Jolles, Samuel N. (father of Róża Maria), 52
Joseph II, emperor, 13–14, 16, 34, 37, 45, 49, 92, 108
Jurasz, Antoni, 146

K
Kalahora, Mattathias, 4n8
Kalahora, Salomon. *See* Calahora, Salomon
Kalmus, Adelle (Ada). *See* Reichenstein, Adelle
Kalmus, Maria. *See* Schneider, Maria
Kapuściński, Józef, 96
Karo, Joseph. *See* Caro, Joseph
Kazantseva, Tetiana, *113*
Kędzierski, Zygmunt, 118
Kelles-Krauz, Janina, 82
Klarfeld, Jakub, 96
Kohn, Józef, 60
Kolischer, Joseph (grandfather of Maurycy Lazarus), 49
Kolischer, Józef, 54
Kolischer, Juliusz, 60
Kolischer, Mindel (grandmother of Maurycy Lazarus), 49
Kolischer, Rosa. *See* Lazarus, Rosa
Korczak, Janusz, 81
Korngold, Regina, 33n69
Korytska-Holub, Yulia, *107*
Kościuszko, Tadeusz, 61
Kremler, Anton, 9n20
Krupiński, Jędrzej, 9n20

L
Lampronti, Isaac, 8n16
Landau, Jan, 137
Landau, Joachim, 60
Lateiner, Matylda, 34, 35
Lazarus, Eleonora (daughter of ML). *See* Diamand, Eleonora
Lazarus, Isaac (brother of ML), 45
Lazarus, Józef (Joseph/Josip) (son of ML), 42n, *70*, 71–72
Lazarus, Feige (grandmother of ML), 49
Lazarus, Fryderyka (daughter of ML), 73, 75, 81–82, 83
Lazarus, Helen (wife of Victor Karl Lazarus, grandson of ML), 72nn93–94
Lazarus, Hermina (daughter of ML). *See* Diamand, Hermina
Lazarus, Hugo (son of ML), 84
Lazarus, Lazar (grandfather of ML), 45, 47, 49
Lazarus, Marcus (uncle of ML), 51
Lazarus, Maurycy (Mojżesz/Moritz/Moriz/Moses), vii, xiii, xiv, 42–43, 45–46, *48*, 49–70, 73, 81, 84–85, 97, 103–4, *106–7*, 109, 113–14, 118, 122, 129, 154, 156
Lazarus, Rachel (sister of ML), 45
Lazarus, Rosa (*née* Kolischer) (mother of ML), 45, 47, *48–49*
Lazarus, Róża Maria (Rosa Marie) (*née* Jolles) (wife of ML), 43, 52–53, 63, 66, 70, 73–74, 81, 84, 97, 122
Lazarus, Simche (father of ML), 45, 47–48, *49*
Lazarus, Sofie (*née* Ergas) (wife of Józef/Joseph/Josip Lazarus, son of ML), 71–72
Lazarus, Victor Karl (grandson of ML), 70, 72n93
Lazarus, Wictoria (daughter of ML), 70n88
Lazarus, ? (son of ML), 70n88
Lehm, Samuel, 145, *146*
Lem, Stanisław Herman, 145n89
Lenkiewicz, Adam, *145*

Leo (Lev), prince, 90
Leon of Modena, 8n16
Levyns'kyi (Levyns'ka), Josefa (*née* Hauser), 114
Levyns'kyi (Lewiński), Ivan (Jan), 43, 114–18
Levyns'kyi, Ivan Sr., *114*
Lewin, Moses, 12
Löffler, Leopold, 103n21
Lustgarten, Waleria, 33n69
Luxemburg, Rosa, 116
Luz, Franciscus de, 9

M
Mahl, Fryderyk Jan, 35
Mahl, Lea (*née* Epstein), 23n48
Mahl, Moses, 23
Malfitano, Giovanni, 75
Maria Theresa, sovereign, 12–13
Mayer, Natan, 64
Mayerhofer, Ernst, 34
Mazur, Dawid 73
Mehler, Koppel, *6*
Mehrer, Henryk (Herschl, Heinrich, Henry), 25nn50-51, *99–102*, 104–6, 133–37
Meisels, Samuel, 140
Menachem, Simcha. *See* DeJona, Emanuel
Mendelssohn, Moses, 49
Metropolis, Nicholas, 119
Metternich, Klemens von, 107
Mieses, Herman, 60
Mikan, Gottfried, 13
Minkiewicz, Witold, 120
Mokłowski, Kazimierz Julian, *98, 103*, 115–18
Mordechai, son of Yitzhak, 92
Morpurgos, medical family, 5
Münz, Marek, *43, 91, 141*
Münzer, Jakub, 142, 147

N
Napoleon Bonaparte, 24
Neumann, John von, 119
Niedziałkowska, Wiktoria, 73
Nüll, Eduard van der, 112

O
Oberländer, Samuel, 147
Oehlenberg (Öhlenberg), Maria, 145
Oettinger, Józef, 16, 17nn36–37, 130
Ogesser, Franz, 9n20
Oppeheimer, Samuel, 131
Ornstein, Jacob Meshulam, rabbi, 92
Ornstein, Sarah, 92

P
Parnas, Emil, 138
Pereira, Adolf, baron, 107
Perl, Emilia, 31
Perl, Joseph, 17n37
Perneuer, François, *10*
Perrot, Georges, 113
Pictorius, Copilius, *6*
Piepes, Jakub, 61
Piepes, Salomon, 25n53
Piłsudska, Aleksandra (*née* Szczerbińska), 79
Piłsudski, Józef, 79
Pirogov, Nikolai, 104, *107*
Pisek, Wilhelm, 133–35, *136*, 144
Podwysocka, Maria, *82*
Popiel, Antoni, 103, *106*
Potocki, Alfred Józef, count, 54

R
Rappaport, Jacob, 17, 20–22, 25, 26n55
Rappaport, Mordechai, 17, 20n38
Rappaport, Moritz (Markus), 17, 26–27, *30*, 34
Rappaport, Nanette (Nina), 25
Rawska, Helena (pseud). *See* Diamand (*née* Lazarus), Hermina
Reich, Alfred, 34n73
Reich, Franciszka (*née* Fuchs), 34
Reichenstein, Adelle (*née* Kalmus), 31, 33
Reichenstein, Marek, 30–31
Rosco-Bogdanowicz, Marian, 53, 55
Rosenberg, Alexander, 147
Rosenberg, Samuel, 12
Rothschild, Anselm Salomon von, baron, 131
Rothschild, Salomon Freiherr von, baron, 131
Rubinstein, Lazar, 96
Ruff, Salomon (Stanisław), 133–34, 144
Rydygier, Ludwik, 134
Rzewuski, W., *130*

S
Samuel bar Meshulam, 4
Sanguszko, Eustachy, prince, 55
Saphier, Jan, *146*
Sapieha, Adam, prince, 55
Sapieha, Władysław, prince, 55
Schaff, Szymon, 56, 66
Schams, Franz, *51*
Schmidt, Friedrich, 112
Schmidt, Wilhelm, 108–9
Schneider, Maria (*née* Kalmus), 31, 32–33
Schneider, Natan Aron, 31, 33n70, 146n92
Schwarz, Arnold, 146
Selzer, Marcin, 147
Semper, Gottfried, 109
Sheptytsky, Andrey, archbishop, 129
Sicardsburg, August Sicard von, 112
Silberstein, Maurycy (Mojżesz Dawid), 96
Skrzyński, Ludwik, 54
Sobieski, Jan, king, 4
Sosnowski, Oskar, 119
Spaventi, Johann, 9n20
Stacherski, Antoni, 131
Stecher von Sebenitz, Ferdinand, 25, 32
Stiassny, Wilhelm, 113, 132
Stroh, Jakub, 96

T
Taubes, Israel, 96
Thurnheim, Samuel, 35
Trębacz, Maurycy, 104

Trzemeski, E., *62, 63, 129*

U
Ulam, Abraham Bernard, 118
Ulam, Cecylia (Czajtel) (*née* Koller), 118
Ulam, Lea Leonia (*née* Caro), 118
Ulam, Michał, *111,112,* 118–120, *121*
Ulam, Stanisław Marcin, 118–19
Ungar, Maximilian, 145n87
Uziel, Abraham, 12

V
Van Swieten, Gerhard, 12

W
Wachtel, Wilhelm, 103–4, *106*
Wallich, Isaac, 8n14
Waltz, Johann, 9n20, 13n27
Waringer, Dina. *See* Epstein, Dina
Waringer, Isaac, 25, 37, 92
Warschauer, Jonatan, 16, 17n36
Weis, Leopold (Weisz, Lipot), *64*
Weinreb, Abraham, 25n53
Welt, Rosa, 31
Wiśniowski, Teofil, 96
Wolf, Aron, 147
Wolf, Salomon, 16, 17n36
Wróblewski, Walery, general, 78, 79n108
Wyczółkowski, Leon, 103n21
Wysłouch, Maria, 73
Wyspiański, Stanisław, 116

Z
Zachariewicz, Alfred, 119
Zachariewicz, Julian, 64, 109, *110,* 113–14
Zimorowicz, Józef Bartołomiej, 91n1
Znamierowska, Maria, *82*

www.ingramcontent.com/pod-product-compliance
Lightning Source LLC
Chambersburg PA
CBHW040844100426
42812CB00014B/2602